Informed Consent
Patient Autonomy and Clinician Beneficence within Health Care
SECOND EDITION

CLINICAL MEDICAL ETHICS

Editors

H. TRISTRAM ENGELHARDT, JR., The Center for Ethics, Medicine and Public Issues, Baylor College of Medicine, Houston, Texas

KEVIN WILDES, S.J., Department of Philosophy, Georgetown University, Washington, D.C.

Editorial Advisory Board

GEORGE J. AGICH, School of Medicine, Southern Illinois University, Springfield, Illinois

DAN W. BROCK, Department of Philosophy, Brown University, Providence, Rhode Island

BARUCH A. BRODY, Center for Ethics, Medicine and Public Issues, Baylor College of Medicine, Houston, Texas

ALLEN E. BUCHANAN, School of Medicine, University of Wisconsin at Madison, Madison, Wisconsin

ANTONIO M. GOTTO, JR., Department of Medicine, Baylor College of Medicine, Houston, Texas

ANGELA R. HOLDER, School of Medicine, Yale University, New Haven, Connecticut

JAY KATZ, Yale Law School, Yale University, New Haven, Connecticut

LORETTA M. KOPELMAN, Department of Medical Humanities, School of Medicine, East Carolina University, Greenville, North Carolina

EDMUND D. PELLEGRINO, Director, Center for Clinical Bioethics, Georgetown University, Washington, D.C.

STEPHEN WEAR, Department of Philosophy, State University of New York at Buffalo, Buffalo, New York

Previous Books in the Series

Informed Consent
Patient Autonomy and Clinician Beneficence within Health Care

SECOND EDITION

Stephen Wear

GEORGETOWN UNIVERSITY PRESS / WASHINGTON, D.C.

Georgetown University Press, Washington, D.C.
© 1998 by Georgetown University Press. All rights reserved
Printed in the United States of America
10 9 8 7 6 5 4 3 2 1   1998
THIS VOLUME IS PRINTED ON ACID-FREE OFFSET BOOK PAPER

Library of Congress Cataloging-in-Publication Data

Wear, Stephen.
    Informed consent: patient autonomy and clinician beneficence
within health care / Stephen Wear. — 2nd ed.
        p.   cm.
    Includes bibliographical references and index.
    1. Informed consent (Medical law).   2. Medical ethics.   I. Title.
    [DNLM: 1. Ethics, Medical.   2. Informed Consent.   3. Patient
Participation.   4. Physician-Patient Relations.   W 50 W362i 1998]
R724.W355   1998
174'.2—dc21
DNLM/DLC
for Library of Congress
ISBN 0-87840-706-5 (paper)   98-15856

To Christa and Cullen,
My wife and son,

And in memory of my grandparents,
Florence Ella and Herbert Spenser Wear

Contents

Preface to the Second Edition

It is now over four years since the first edition of this book was published and, one might say, "Much has changed while much has stayed the same." The sources of change are various. I have been honored by a number of detailed reviews of this work by others in the field.[1] Numerous colleagues, in Buffalo and elsewhere, have shared their thoughts with me about this work and its subject matter. Most significantly, a couple of years back my book was the focus of a reading group of local scholars and clinicians where it was reviewed, roughly a chapter per meeting, and all sorts of differences of emphasis as well as view were presented to me. In fact, to the extent that this second edition improves on its predecessor, these colleagues should be acknowledged and thanked: Jack Freer, M.D.; Jan Harszlak, M.A.; Charles Jack, M.A.; Paul Johnson, Ph.D.; Janet Kaye, J.D.; Bogda Koczwara, M.D.; Dan Lazenski, J.D.; Sue LaGaipa, R.N., M.A.; Gerald Logue, M.D.; Sherrie Lyons, Ph.D.; Tim Madigan; Adrianne McEvoy; James Moran, Ph.D.; Daniel Pollock, Ph.D.; Ann Poutler; Carolyn Siegel; and Anthony Szczygiel, J.D.

I am sure, however, that I am not the first author who has been torn between the tendency to try to "improve on the original" in a subsequent edition of a work and the feeling that the initial product has its own "rights," as it were, and changes should be sparing.

For those especially who took the time to read the original edition, I hope it will be sufficient here to simply say that I eventually resolved the preceding tension as follows: major substantive changes have not been made to this work. It contains the same basic argument, in roughly the same form and sequence as the first edition; its main conclusions also remain the same. What is different is my attempt, particularly by responding to the questions and criticisms of colleagues, to remove unclarity and confusion in the text, as well as to make it as clear as possible what any given section is attempting to investigate or prove.

One particular issue especially called for my renewed attention in this edition—namely, the reasons and sense for my emphasis on an event model of informed consent within a larger process. This is so as I have found that although I intended to emphasize both the event and the process characteristics of informed consent, my presentation tended to fall too heavily on the event aspect of it, engendering significant misunderstanding of my sense of and concern for its process aspect. Moreover, I did find myself reconceiving this dual event-process model of informed consent in certain ways and felt forced to rectify certain deficiencies in my original account, particularly in response to the suggestions of colleagues.

Finally, one subsection is wholly new to this second edition—namely, the discussion under the heading of "the clinician's discretion" in the final, ninth chapter. This section renders more explicit and detailed my earlier view that considerable variability exists, from patient to patient, and case to case, regarding how significant, or not, the various goods and values that informed consent might pursue actually will be. Given such variability, including the fact that some potential values may simply not be at stake in certain cases—for example, the need for a detailed actual understanding on the patient's part—effective clinical management requires a wide range of discretion on the part of clinicians. This specific discussion is provided by reference to Howard Brody's work, specifically to his extended remarks about the whole issue of physician power, as well as his transparency model of informed consent. In both regards, Brody not only offers somewhat alternate views to those of this work, but also casts certain issues in a particularly relevant fashion. And, as I found myself searching for a way to make certain matters clearer in this edition, Brody's thought eventually emerged as the best and most efficient foil to attempt this, in large part as we agree on so much.

In sum, all the concerns operative in the original introduction remain in force, as do my views on the facts and clinical realities that must be attended to in developing a clinically nuanced and effective model of informed consent, particularly as the "management tool" that I sought to originally articulate.

NOTE

1. Jonathan Moreno (SUNY Health Science Center, Brooklyn) in *Healthcare Ethics Committee Forum* 6, no. 5 (September 1994): 323–25; Joanna Pasek (University College, London, England) in *Journal of Medical Ethics* 21, no. 2 (April 1995): 119–20; Arthur Caplan (University of Pennsylvania) in *Journal of the American Geriatrics Association* 43, no. 12 (December 1995): 3–5; Andrew Crowden (Deakin University, Australia) in *Bioethics* 10, no. 1 (1996): 83–86; Andrew Lustig (Institute of Religion, Texas Medical Center) in *Journal of Medicine and Philosophy* 21 (1996): 101–9; Vivienne Nathanson (British Medical Association, London) in *International Digest of Health Legislation* 47, no. 2 (1996): 273–75.

Acknowledgments

I would like to express my deep gratitude to the following colleagues who provided me with detailed critical reactions to this manuscript: H. Tristram Engelhardt, Jr., Ph.D., M.D.; George Khushf, Ph.D.; Susan LaGaipa, M.S., R.N.; Laurence McCullough, Ph.D.; Jonathan Moreno, Ph.D.; E. Haavi Morreim, Ph.D.; Benjamin Phillips, M.S., R.N.; and Stuart Spicker, Ph.D.

A parallel debt should also be acknowledged to my clinical colleagues in the Buffalo medical community who helped me gain insight into the realities of clinical medicine. John Banas, M.D.; William Coles, M.D.; Jack Freer, M.D.; and Paul Katz, M.D., merit special thanks in this regard. Norman Chassin, M.D., also deserves singling out, especially for his extended and patient attempt to help me see that the tradition of physician beneficence was truly worthy of the name, however much we may continue to quarrel about its specific pronouncements. Special thanks are also due to Gerald Logue, M.D., and Paul Davis, M.D., who encouraged and supported me in my work in clinical medicine as an ethics consultant, and provided me with access to their patients and staff.

Finally, a special note of appreciation is due to H. Tristram Engelhardt, Jr., Ph.D., M.D., and Laurence McCullough, Ph.D., not only for their assistance with this book, but especially for their sustained support, encouragement, understanding, and friendship over the years.

Notice

Except in the instance of cases that have been reported in the public media or have become public through court hearings, all identifiable information used in case examples has been changed, and the structure of the case example altered, so as not to identify the individuals involved. Instead, case examples have been constructed out of numerous clinical experiences so as to illustrate a general problem in bioethics, health care delivery, or health care policy. Any similarity to actual individuals living or dead is purely coincidental.

Also, though legal cases and principles are examined in this volume, there is no intention to provide legal advice. For legal advice there is no substitute for directly consulting the legal profession.

Introduction

The first issue a book on informed consent should address is why it was written at all. Of all the current pressing topics in biomedical ethics, whether we refer to the issue of abortion, to the controversies surrounding access to health care, or to the myriad dilemmas ingredient in the area of death and dying, informed consent seems to pale as an issue. Equally, it would seem that agreement has long since been reached on the ethical necessity for the informed consent of competent patients, indicating that this is no longer a controversial issue. The law is absolutely clear about this, and so are most bioethicists. Finally, at least from the perspective of practicing clinicians, the intended audience of this series, the most that might be desired is an explanation of the law on informed consent, particularly regarding how to honor its requirements (or avoid its sanctions) at the bedside. But such "cookbook" approaches to informed consent have been offered.[1] Another is hardly needed.

This book does not offer legal advice. As we shall see, there is, in fact, no clear single, settled law regarding informed consent to explicate. Rather, legal pronouncements on and criteria for informed consent vary from state to state in the United States (where the law on informed consent is the most highly evolved). Equally, these "guidelines" often exist only within the context of specific legal cases, not in formal statutes, so that their interpretation will also have to attend to similarities or differences among various individual precedents. Further, legal guidelines regarding informed consent range from the quite specific and complex in some countries to a total absence of any legal insistence upon it in others, particularly in the third world and in totalitarian countries. Thus for the practicing clinician who is curious about "the law" regarding informed consent there is no substitute for consulting a legal colleague in the particular jurisdiction in which he practices.[2]

1

However, with respect to the perception that the nature of informed consent has already been sufficiently articulated in the past, and agreement gained regarding it, this work proceeds from the opposing conviction that neither closure nor adequate statement has yet been achieved. This is so because, however much the ethical necessity of informed consent is apparent to its proponents, many of those who must provide informed consent to patients—namely, practicing clinicians—are at best lukewarm about it. Equally, clinicians are often unclear about what it should actually amount to at the bedside, even when they are generically committed to it. Many practicing clinicians also harbor strong doubts about both the need for it, at least in every instance of the institution of therapy, and the appropriateness of the assumptions that underlie it—for example, that most competent patients are ready, willing, and able to "participate in medical decision-making," as the proponents of informed consent claim. However much the bioethicists and lawyers may consider the issue of informed consent to be beyond debate, many of those who must provide it remain quite unconvinced (and, crucially, uncommitted to it). Mention informed consent to a clinician and my experience is that you are more likely to get a groan, as well as talk about the "myth of informed consent." Seldom will one encounter a clinician who sees informed consent as simply a useful tool for medical management. This book explores and evaluates the nature and grounds of such clinician skepticism, and responds by offering a cogent, clinically realistic model of informed consent.

This work also proceeds in terms of the conviction that informed consent does not "pale" in comparison to other current issues in bioethics. First, it is eminently clear to this author that of all the elements ingredient in the reorientation that has occurred in medical ethics over the past couple of decades, the informed consent doctrine is potentially the most profound and far-reaching. Informed consent is aimed at both enabling and empowering a patient population that has traditionally been largely mute and powerless in the face of medical expertise and authority (Katz, 1984). By placing obligations regarding informed consent on health care providers, the doctrine mandates the provision of information upon which patients can fashion their own views and decisions about the manner of their care. Equally, patients are given the power to enforce their decisions, a power now enshrined as the right to refuse treatment. Informed consent is thus the cutting edge of the patient autonomy movement. Through it, proponents of autonomy-based medical ethics have proceeded far beyond concerns about extraordinary cases to the advocacy of a general restructuring of the form of every encounter between patient and clinician. But—and here is the rub—absent a cogent and clinically effective tool for respecting and enhancing patient autonomy, such refusals become suspect, and uncommitted clinicians provide ineffective rituals; this leaves the respect vacuous and the enhancement absent. In the end, the "new ethos of patient autonomy" runs the risk of being no more than the latest set of the "emperor's new clothes."

This book offers a cogent and realistic model of informed consent to practicing clinicians and seeks especially to present it as a useful tool for medical management. To accomplish this, it responds directly to the profound differences of opinion regarding informed consent that exist between its proponents and many clinicians. As a philosopher functioning within medical school and clinical settings for two decades, this author has come to see important truths and values on both sides. As the proponents of informed consent argue, it is clear that the "silent world of doctor and patient," which the physician Jay Katz has described, challenges some of the most fundamental convictions of a free society (Katz, 1984). There can be no freedom, no personal control of one's life, in an arena where knowledge and power are systematically withheld by others. Detractors from informed consent, however, have forcefully replied that, whatever strides the medical consumer movement has made among the healthy and educated, the sick still generally come to their physicians for expertise and reassurance, not knowledge and power. They want to be fixed and reassured, not educated and forced to make decisions about matters with which they are quite unfamiliar.

The gulf here is deep once one moves beyond the surfaces and the rituals that are played out upon them. This book aims to fashion a compromise between these two apparently opposing and mutually exclusive views on the doctrine of informed consent. This author finds truth and insight on both sides, but also error and misconception. Though often too theoretical and inattentive to practical realities, the proponents of informed consent have articulated the foundations of a strong case for the need for informed consent—namely, that too many important goods and values are lost in its absence (or by its "ritualistic provision"). As to its clinician detractors, though some of them throw the baby out with the bathwater, their criticisms of the doctrine of informed consent as unrealistic, ineffective, and, in effect, unintelligible, are often forceful and cogent, and merit detailed reply. Informed consent is not a myth, as some would have it, for the simple reason that too many important values ride on it for us to allow it to be a myth (see chapter 4 in this regard). However, as articulated in both the law and the ethics literature, informed consent is not yet adequately fashioned to be successfully grafted onto the heart of clinical practice. As a result, in practice, it is too often little more than a ritual, offered grudgingly and without conviction by clinicians.

The overall aim of this book is to fashion a comprehensive sense of informed consent as an effective, efficient, and needed tool for medical management. Such a practical enterprise, however, will first necessitate an extended tour of the insights and arguments of its proponents and critics toward two basic ends: (1) to identify those goods and values that informed consent can justifiably pursue, and (2) to place and inform such a pursuit within the context of those clinical realities that have made many clinicians rather skeptical about both the potential effectiveness of and the need for such a pursuit. Toward such a perspective on informed consent, the first part of this work, entitled "The Sources of a Model of Informed Consent," will proceed through the following stages. The first chapter will identify the essentials of the evolved legal doctrine of informed consent, particularly toward providing us with a sense of the issues such a model must speak to and what its structure and content might be. Given the aforementioned variations across jurisdictions and countries, this legal doctrine will at best be a useful "fiction," useful both by providing an initial model from which we can proceed, and by supplying a sense of what the law, even in its most highly evolved form, does *and* does not speak to. We will find that the "legal doctrine" generates more questions and controversies than it solves, particularly as we move from what might be legally mandated to what is clinically and ethically feasible and appropriate.

This initial result will necessitate a more wide-ranging analysis of the debate over informed consent and patient autonomy, which will begin in the second chapter, "The New Ethos of Patient Autonomy." This chapter will further specify and corroborate the claim that both sides should be seen as having truth and insight, as well as misconceptions and error, in their formulations and arguments. Chapter 3 will then depart from the more legalistic and theoretical forms of its two predecessors and consider "The Clinical Experience of Patient Autonomy and Informed Consent." This chapter will analyze the common perspective and experience of clinicians regarding informed consent, as well as provide a general review of relevant empirical studies. The fourth and final chapter of this first part, entitled "The Potential Benefits of Informed Consent," will then identify precisely the goods and values informed consent can capture if understood and realistically pursued in a clinically and ethically sound fashion. This chapter, in sum, will supply the argument that there are too many important goods and values at stake for us either to maintain a skeptical approach to informed consent or to pursue it by means of some inflexible ritual. The second part of this work (chapters 5 through 9) will then proceed to articulate an ethically and clinically cogent and realistic model of informed consent, generated out of and informed by the sources articulated in these first four chapters.

One final word of introduction: The following conviction should be seen as seminal to and operant throughout this work: that the doctrine of informed consent, as currently articulated in the law and the bioethics literature, suffers from a substantially ritualistic and rhetorical character that both lessens its effectiveness and makes it presume to provide benefits that it often fails to accomplish. In large part, this is so because this doctrine remains uncalibrated to the realities and variables within clinical medicine. The final aim of this work will thus be to go beyond the rhetoric and provide the realism requisite for establishing informed consent as an effective and needed tool for medical management. The practicing clinician should understand that we are about to discuss a basic aspect of the provision of good medical care, no more, and no less.

NOTES

1. The most detailed of such offerings is Rozovsky, 1984. It provides both conceptual analysis of legal principles and guidance regarding specific interventions and consent situations.

2. Regarding the use of the singular indefinite pronoun here, I will follow the lead of my predecessor in this series, E. Haavi Morreim, who states: "Throughout this volume I will observe the somewhat old-fashioned but still correct custom of using the masculine pronoun in its gender-neutral form to stand as the singular indefinite pronoun (see Shertzer, 1986, p. 20). To substitute plural pronouns such as 'they' or 'their' is incorrect; consistently using the feminine pronoun instead of the masculine is no less biased; and alternating between the two seems awkward and contrived." Morreim, 1995, p. 7.

PART I

The Sources of
a Model of
Informed Consent

1

The Legal Doctrine of Informed Consent

Clinicians often respond to ethical issues by first inquiring as to what the relevant law dictates. The instinct is a prudent one. It is not very sensible to discuss ethical options that the law prohibits, or attempt to fashion a response when the law has already provided one and insists upon it.

As already noted, however, the law regarding informed consent varies across jurisdictions and countries, so in a global sense there is no single and settled sense of the law to explicate, not even on the level of basic principles and criteria. What will now be provided, instead, will be a general portrait of the law on informed consent in the United States, where a legal view of informed consent is the most highly evolved. Even this, however, will remain at most a useful fiction, as jurisdictions within the United States provide different formulations of key principles and criteria. In what follows, then, reference to the "legal doctrine" on informed consent should be received as referring to just such a fiction which, however useful for our purposes here, is no substitute for a detailed sense of the law on informed consent in any specific jurisdiction.

One of the uses of the fictitious "legal doctrine of informed consent" presented here will be to gain a first approximation of what a model of informed consent might look like—that is, what are its goals and agendas, its operating principles and criteria, and what types of information it tends to insist on conveying. Presentation of this "legal doctrine" will also allow us to investigate whether the law provides an ethically and clinically adequate model of informed consent—that is, whether the law comprehensively identifies and keys to the proper goals and agendas, whether its methodology and criteria appear adequate to capture these goals, and whether its underlying assumptions are clinically realistic. Finally, this chapter will enable us to identify ways in which the legal doctrine of informed consent simply does *not* speak to issues and agendas that a clinically and ethically satisfactory model must address. We should keep in mind that the law often tends to speak, at most, to what one might see as minimally necessary, as opposed to ethically sufficient, in a given area.

THE GOALS AND SOURCES OF THE
LEGAL DOCTRINE OF INFORMED CONSENT

In a nutshell, a legally valid informed consent should instruct the patient regarding (1) the problem or diagnosis for which further investigation or intervention is proposed, (2) the recommended intervention coupled with the significant benefits and risks attendant to it, (3) the results or prognosis if no intervention is attempted, and (4) any significant alternative modalities with their attendant risks and benefits. Further, all competent patients must receive such information about any diagnostic or therapeutic intervention except in situations where (1) the patient is threatened with serious harm or death if the intervention is not immediately provided (the *emergency exception*), or (2) the patient voluntarily gives up the right to be so informed and consents, in advance, to what the physician considers the appropriate form of action (the *waiver exception*), or (3) the physician has sufficient reason to believe that disclosure itself would cause serious physical or psychological harm to the patient (the *"therapeutic privilege" exception*). Concerning which patients are competent (and thus entitled) to give an informed consent, such competence should be presumed unless sufficient reasons to the contrary are identified—for example, gross mental deficits or incapacity. And, finally, all this should occur without any coercion or manipulation that undermines the patient's ability to choose.

The preceding may seem straightforward enough, but numerous issues quickly arise as one reflects further. (1) Even though the types of information are clear, we also need more specific criteria for determining which information should actually be disclosed within a given type. This is particularly the case when one gets to the disclosure of the risks of an intervention, because, as reference to any drug insert advises us, the *possible* risks of any intervention are usually quite numerous. So some selection criteria regarding the main or most significant risks are essential, lest risk disclosure degenerate into an undifferentiated list that tends to produce information overload rather than insight in the patient. (2) We need to know what specific criteria are available to determine whether one of the three exceptions to informed consent may be legitimately appealed to in a given case; without clear and specific definition, exceptions tend to destroy the rule. (3) An operational definition of competence is required so that one can determine who shall or should not be offered an informed consent—that is, what are "sufficient reasons" to abandon the mandated presumption of competence in a given case? (4) Finally, for our own broader purposes, as well as toward understanding the legal doctrine, we need a clearer sense of the goals and agendas that the law is pursuing by means of this doctrine and, then, a sense of how well or poorly it meets them. Let us begin by addressing this last issue, particularly in terms of the development of the law regarding informed consent: What is the law trying to accomplish by means of informed consent?[1]

Prior to the twentieth century, some precedents showed concern for issues such as whether the patient had consented to a procedure (without concern for the provision of any information), whether physicians are obliged to alert patients to basic risks of a proposed treatment, and whether fraud had occurred in the case of a physician's representation of a patient's problem (Faden and Beauchamp, 1986, pp. 114–25). In the past these sorts of issues were usually resolved by referring to the customary practice of members of the medical profession. In effect, the traditional response to many of our questions was that the medical profession itself was the legally recognized source of guidelines and criteria, not specific legal principles and agendas.

Reliance on the customary practice of the medical profession— that is, on professional standards—surely makes things simpler for the clinician, at least to the extent that an individual clinician shares a common training, experience, and perspective with his peers, and should have a general sense of what is customary. The clinician is thus not also obliged to attempt to fathom the different languages, agendas, and formulations of the legal profession. Ironically, as Flexner's reforms of medical education made such a common experience and perspective among clinicians more of a reality, the law tended to shift away from a solely professional standard.

In the early twentieth century, certain principles and agendas that had long been basic to the law but less central to medical practice began to come to the fore in judicial determinations regarding patient consent and patient-physician interactions. Most basic, at first glance, was the common law's traditional concern for the "bodily integrity of the individual," in effect a concern for patient "self-determination," which at least requires patient consent to treatment, however uninformed.[2] But other legal concerns and agendas also began to assert themselves: (1) the law's prescription against battery—that is, the "unauthorized touching" of one individual by another (Faden and Beauchamp, 1986, pp. 120–22); (2) tort law's concern about the infliction of physical and emotional harm, and legal mechanisms for compensation (Faden and Beauchamp, 1986, pp. 125–32), and (3) the constitutional concern for the individual's privacy, his right to be left alone.[3]

The specific history of the modern emergence of such concerns into matters traditionally seen as relating to medical custom and expertise is quite controversial among legal scholars (Faden and Beauchamp, 1986, pp. 53–60). The controversy relates particularly to which principle or branch of law is governing. One option here is to emphasize patient self-determination, which many of the decisions do, at least rhetorically.[4] But strong argument has been advanced that the principle of self-determination has not been the dominant force behind the development of the legal doctrine.[5] Had it been so, courts would have developed more specific disclosure requirements and guidelines. They also would have been much more concerned about the most effective ways to enhance understanding and fight against ritualistic disclosures that barely satisfy the letter, much less the spirit, of such a legal principle. Another way to put this is that if courts were truly concerned about patient self-determination, then an offense against it—for example, not adequately informing a patient—would in and of itself be treated as an actionable harm, even if no other physical or emotional harm occurred. A lack of *informed* consent could be considered and penalized as a battery, an unauthorized touching, even if a bare consent had been obtained and the intervention was medically successful.

But such developments have not occurred. A lack of informed consent has been actionable, and damages awarded, *only when* its absence could be shown to have caused some *other* emotional or physical harm. By way of example, if a patient was not told of the risk of death from general anesthesia, and death did *not* occur, damages would not be awarded simply for the affront to patient self-determination. If, however, such a result did occur, and it could be proved that the patient would not have undergone the procedure had he known of that risk, then damages would be awarded for the injury, even if it was a foreseeable risk of the intervention and no other malpractice was involved. In sum, the complete lack of consent is actionable as a battery, an inadequate consent is actionable only if some emotional or physical injury also resulted, but there is no legal action for an inadequate provision of information per se.

This state of affairs may not seem disconcerting to clinicians, particularly given the current malpractice climate, in that damages are awarded only if there are actual emotional or physical injuries, not simply if an adequate informed consent is lacking in a situation where treatment is otherwise benign or successful. But to those who are concerned that patient self-determination itself be protected *and* fostered in clinical medicine, and who see a lack of an informed consent as a serious affront and harm to a patient's liberty and privacy, all this may be regrettable. For our purposes, the significance of the preceding is that much of the development of the legal doctrine of informed consent has instead occurred within the context of tort law, in malpractice actions.

The reason why this result is unfortunate is *not* that the law has failed to pursue a positive account of informed consent, particularly as a vehicle for protecting and enhancing patient self-determination. It would arguably be inappropriate to use the law for such a task, in effect using it as a vehicle to modify and micromanage clinician behavior. I submit, without argument at this point, that the valid agendas of informed consent will only be met by clinicians who are sold on and committed to the enterprise. The law can neither accurately calibrate nor sufficiently motivate the necessary behaviors by itself. It can, at most, mandate minimal requirements. Such minimal requirements then need ethical supplementation and support, lacking which they tend to produce ineffective informed consent rituals,[6] as many feel has been the actual result—for example, when clinicians hyperinform patients to the point of information overload to guard against a charge of inadequate disclosure.

Our focus should regard the ethical character and opportunities of informed consent, not how it was flawed in cases where negative outcomes also occurred. Part of the problem with the legal doctrine is that informed consent thus comes to be perceived, by both patients and physicians, as involving threats to which the physician must respond, not as a vehicle for respecting and promoting patient self-determination and enhancing the patient-physician dialogue. Equally, the sort of guidance and standards that a court might offer in evaluating a suit for damages is not necessarily going to be the same as if it were asked to speak to how informed consent could best protect and enhance patient self-determination. Not that, as I have suggested, we would want to encourage the courts to pursue such a goal. Rather, it must be realized, the law's actual working agendas have been narrower and, in important ways, different from the positive concerns regarding self-determination. But let us move on to the specific guidance that the law does offer regarding our various concerns, concurrently reflecting upon whether its guidance is clinically and ethically adequate.

ELEMENTS OF THE LEGAL DOCTRINE

In terms of the preceding analysis, we should distinguish two sources of explanation regarding the elements of the legal doctrine: (1) the more generic, rhetorical principles to which the law appeals (e.g., patient self-determination) and (2) the more specific guidelines that have arisen largely within the context of tort law regarding malpractice actions. The latter source addresses the specific task of deciding whether damages are due, at least in part, because the patient was not adequately informed of a potential risk that subsequently occurred. It may also be concerned with whether the patient was, in fact, competent to consent, whether fraud or duress biased and invalidated his consent, or whether valid exceptions to informed consent were present, as, for example, in an emergency situation.

Competence to Consent

Competence to consent is to be presumed in most cases, and the burden of proof lies with the one who believes a given patient to be incompetent. This burden obviously is met in situations of coma and gross psychopathology. But the issue is often quite unclear *clinically*. Illness is often accompanied by factors such as fear, stress, pain, the effects of the treatment (e.g., drugs), or the effects of the disease (e.g., lessened oxygenation of the brain due to pulmonary deficits). And such factors tend to diminish a patient's ability to understand and make decisions.

Such factors, though they often trouble the clinician's assessment of competence, are given little recognition in the law. This may, in part, be due to the lack of clinical experience of lawyers, in that they are unfamiliar with such factors, especially their prevalence and variability in patients. They often fail to see that competence, in the functional sense of the ability to understand information and make decisions, must be seen as a *spectrum*, ranging broadly from the impressively knowledgeable and decisive patient to the patient who gives no sign of coherent response. But other factors have contributed to the law's insistence on the presumption of competence. (1) In our legal system high priority is given to freedom and self-determination; the concern would thus be that if such diminishing factors are given too large a significance, competence would be questioned too often. (2) In our society we are free to make many decisions, some quite important (e.g., making a will), and competence should usually be neither questioned nor assessed. This insight may well have fueled both the presumption in favor of competence and the sense of it as a threshold concept—that one is either competent or not, and that the variations on either side should be ignored, at least when deciding who is to receive an informed consent. (3) There is a recognition that decisions that appear to others to be unwise, tragic, or foolish must be acceptable as part and parcel of our status as free men and women. In sum, if we attempt to be overly protective in response to the possibility of "bad choices," or "insufficient" patient competence, freedom tends to evaporate in the process. Clinical naivete may have made it easier for the law to be comfortable with the idea of simply presuming patient competence. One should recognize, however, that the law has other important concerns in this area, and would still probably insist on this presumption, even in the face of the realities that trouble clinicians.

Other developments in the law and in medicine may also lie behind this strong presumption in favor of competence. In the 1960s, serious controversy arose within psychiatry, and concurrently in the law, over the treatment of the mentally ill and the issue of involuntary commitment. Leaving aside whether the pendulum has swung too far, it now seems fair to say that traditional, quite expansive views on who is incompetent and committable have been replaced by a broad concern, in both psychiatry and the law, to "mainstream" the mentally ill and developmentally disabled out into the community where they can enjoy the freedoms of the rest of us.[7] This commitment has been extended to all patients in the form of a quite *low-threshold* view of competence. Even the presence of mental illness does not necessarily prove incompetence to consent to or refuse treatment. In an increasing number of jurisdictions, even involuntarily committed patients are still seen as potentially able to consent to or refuse specific treatment modalities (Rozovsky, 1984, pp. 337–73). Forceful attacks by clinicians on the effects of such a view (one article is aptly entitled "Dying with Your Rights On" [Treffert, 1974]) have had little effect to the contrary.

The application of such a low-threshold view to day-to-day assessments of competency follows directly. Given that incompetency is, strictly speaking, a judicial, *not* a medical, determination, and given that patients of borderline competence are usually evaluated by psychiatrists, persons with marginal capacities to understand and make decisions are, in practice, treated as competent to consent. Further, given that a history of or the presence of mental illness is not, per se, proof of incompetency, the issue has increasingly come to be evaluated within the context of specific treatment decisions, not any global decision-making capacity (Appelbaum, 1987, pp. 82–87). This development is in line with the law in other areas where an individual with a given level of capacity might be deemed capable of making some decisions, but not others—for example, to execute a simple will but not a complex one (Wear, 1980, pp. 295–97).

The current tendency, then, is to hold that competence or capacity to consent should be assessed individually in terms of the situation and decision at hand—in other words, is the patient capable of understanding and making decisions about his immediate situation and prospects? This much seems clear and currently dominant in the law.

But further questions arise. Should the clinician then assess every patient's understanding of the situation and choice at hand? Aside from not being feasible as a matter of time, such an assessment is not required. The law has clearly stopped at requiring disclosure by physicians, without insisting on a further evaluation of how well it was received. In effect, the presumption of competency also allows one to presume that the disclosure was adequately received by the patient. Will the clinician be protected from suit by a patient who later claims he was incompetent at the time? No such protection is available, and although it would be up to the patient to prove it, one would suspect that a history of mental illness might well be part of a patient-plaintiff's argument. A judicial determination, or a psychiatric consult, could provide protection for the clinician in this regard, but, of course, neither can be pursued in most cases. Is the threat of liability on the ground of incompetence substantial? Few successful suits seem to turn mainly on it, but the jeopardy is still abstractly present in the absence of clear clinical standards or guidelines.

The law thus arguably provides insufficient guidance here since it supplies a generic presumption rather than specific clinical criteria for assessing competence. The law, however, has its reasons for not opening what has been referred to as the "Pandora's box" of competence (Roth et al., 1977, p. 282), chiefly that excessive assessment and monitoring of the competence of individual patients would tend to undermine freedom. We will clearly need to spend more time with the options in this regard later (see chapter 7 particularly). But, given that competence to consent is to be raised at the level of the patient's grasp of his individual situation and prospects, the next issue must regard what information must be disclosed, according to the law, about such factors.

Disclosure

The law is quite clear regarding the *types* of information to be disclosed: the problem or diagnosis, the recommended treatment as well as alternate modalities, with their significant risks and benefits, and the prognosis if no treatment is pursued. The law is equally concerned that the communication (and any consent forms) be in lay, not technical terms, that any language barriers be responded to, and that the scope and limits of the intervention be made explicit.

The clinical insufficiency of such guidelines quickly emerges, however, as soon as we inquire as to the level of detail that must be supplied regarding the preceding types of information. Anyone familiar with a drug package insert or a listing for a given drug in the Physician's Desk Reference knows that selection is necessary. To simply parrot the whole list of risks and complications would give the patient no sense of their relative significance, and be more likely to produce information overload than understanding.

Three different standards have had currency for determining which information should be disclosed: (1) the *professional* standard, where the current disclosure practices of the profession itself dictate— in other words, the duty to disclose "is limited to those disclosures which a reasonable medical practitioner would make under the same or similar circumstances";[8] (2) the *reasonable person* standard, where the duty to disclose is dictated by what the "average reasonable person" would deem relevant or material to the decision at hand;[9] and (3) the *subjective* standard, which allows room for the idiosyncratic views and character of the individual patient in determining disclosure.[10]

The law has been reasonably fair, if not sufficiently specific, in choosing among these standards. For one thing, the subjective standard has been arguably utilized in a few court decisions but is mainly a "creature of legal commentary rather than case law" (Faden and Beauchamp, 1986, pp. 33–34 and note 34). Aside from placing physicians in jeopardy to self-serving hindsight or bitterness by patients, it also would call for a degree of familiarity with and insight into the patient's views and values that no physician could possibly be expected to have. If the patient has certain special concerns or agendas, he can raise them. But surely the physician cannot be expected to guess what these agendas and concerns are beforehand or take the time to ferret them out. Second, of the various states, a majority still hold (Faden and Beauchamp, 1986, p. 31 and note 15), by precedent or statute, to a *professional* standard of disclosure, and even when a reasonable person standard is guiding, it is still for the plaintiff to prove that disclosure was insufficient to it.[11] Thus, on either the professional or reasonable person standard, the burden of proof lies with the patient to show that disclosure was inadequate *and* (crucially, since a malpractice suit is the context) that the undisclosed information was a *proximate cause* of the harm or injury. To be a proximate cause, it must be proven that the patient would not have consented to the intervention in the first place had he been adequately informed of the missing information (Faden and Beauchamp, 1986, pp. 34–35).

Whether proximate cause is present is for lawyers to dispute and juries to decide. The overriding issue at this juncture is how the clinician can provide a legally *and* ethically valid disclosure *before the fact*, rather than defend against its absence later. The preceding helps very little in this regard. In fact, by itself, it tends to hurt: uncertainty in the area of which standard is operative, or how it will be applied or interpreted, also tends to make clinicians defensive and hence err on the side of hyperinforming patients, not on the side of sensitive and flexible approaches. If the physician is practicing in a state that emphasizes the professional standard, matters would seem clearer: one only has to be aware of what one's colleagues are doing, not guess what a hypothetical "reasonable person" would consider significant. With an increasing number of physicians going to exorbitant lengths in this regard, however—for example, using elaborate consent forms, videotaping consent sessions, and overinforming "just to be safe"—one at least needs to worry about whether the patient-plaintiff will call on a clinical colleague of the hyperinforming variety. Equally, when the standard is that of the "reasonable person," this is abstract and arbitrary enough—particularly for a jury that is made acutely aware of the plaintiff's injuries by his attorney—that no one in the courtroom may be able to imagine consenting to such a procedure.

One should not overstate the difficulties here, though, as certain rules of thumb are available. As Miller puts it, "whether a risk is material is primarily a function of the likelihood of its occurrence and the severity of the injury it threatens to cause" (Miller and Willner, 1974, p. 965). Thus, minor but common complications, and dire but rare ones, merit disclosure as well as those with average degrees of both frequency and severity.

But an issue of fundamental ethical and clinical moment lurks in the wings here. One may well be forced to decide, in a given case as well as regarding one's habitual practice, between two very conflicting issues: (1) how much should one hyperinform the patient about remote risks or complications to be safe in case a suit later occurs and (2) at what point does disclosure become so detailed and complex that the essential decision at hand is obscured and the patient is overwhelmed rather than edified by the information provided? In sum, the "safe" course of hyperinforming may well be counterproductive to the goal of enhancing patient autonomy; and the course that tends to pursue such an enhancement, by sticking to the "essentials," will correspondingly increase the physician's jeopardy. I submit that it is especially here that the tort basis of much of the legal doctrine directly conflicts and undermines the social policy agendas to which it otherwise expresses allegiance.[12]

Evaluation and Consent

The law has given much less attention to the process by which the patient evaluates the information disclosed, deliberates about its significance within a life unique in its aspirations, experiences, and personal values, and then reaches a decision. Not surprisingly, what scant attention there is in the law to this area concerns physician behaviors that clearly undermine such processes (e.g., fraud, coercion, and manipulation) and biased presentations of the nature of the decision at hand. Aside from blatant assaults on such processes, however, the law's perspective is similar to the one it has on competency. That is, we should *presume* that most patients are sufficiently capable of performing such evaluative and deliberative tasks, if only they are given sufficient information.[13] But from a clinical perspective, such a presumption is particularly questionable. Grasping bits of information is one thing; we might analogize this to a test where specific questions call for specific, short, word or phrase answers. Evaluating the data presented, however, seems much more difficult, for one must first prioritize and relativize it to one's personal circumstance. The patient must then attempt to array all this as a coherent fabric from which a specific decision can be generated. The analogy here would be to the student who is assigned a complex theme or topic on which he must write a balanced essay arguing for a single course of action, which would be, for most of us, a much more precarious and difficult enterprise. If we add to this distinction the previous concern with factors that diminish sick people's mental abilities, and recognize the basic reality that all such information comes wrapped in uncertainties and probabilities that are essential to its meaning and significance, then the task appears even more challenging. Finally, given that the more important a decision is, the more complex it will often be, medically and existentially, then the enterprise of empowering and enabling the patient to participate meaningfully in medical decision making appears all the more precarious. And the law captures very little of this underlying complexity.

We are thus again faced with the law's failing to provide for, or even recognize, clinical realities of fundamental moment. The law has not addressed such complex and precarious matters but merely highlights obvious and blatant assaults on it (e.g., coercion and manipulation). And we are thus, again, left with some direction as to how not to run afoul of the law, but little is provided, in a positive way, concerning what constitutes an ethically satisfactory informed consent. We are also left wondering whether it is realistic to presume that most patients can truly accomplish the task involved, especially if we are speaking of the "essay mode" of patient participation in medical decision making.

Exceptions to the Rule

There are three general exceptions to the rule of gaining informed consent from *competent* patients: the emergency exception, the waiver exception (where the patient gives up the right to be informed), and the exception based on therapeutic privilege (where informing could itself somehow cause significant harm to the patient). Some jurisdictions also countenance not informing patients of "commonly known" risks (Rozovsky, 1984, pp. 66–68), but this exception does not seem to merit consideration as common clinical experience clearly suggests that many patients are woefully ignorant of all matters medical and thus no common knowledge should be assumed.

The Emergency Exception

In general, a physician may render treatment in an emergency. Consent is held to be presumed, given the assumption that most patients would want to be treated in similar circumstances. In the ideal instance, treatment may proceed without having obtained an informed consent if (1) there is a clear, immediate, and serious threat to life and limb, (2) the time it would take to gain an informed consent would seriously jeopardize the patient's hope of recovery (or increase mortality and morbidity), and (3) the patient exhibits factors that may well be undermining his competence to consent, such as shock, hypoxia, or blood loss.[14] To the extent that the case at hand recedes from this tripartite ideal, however, the law's guidance tends to evaporate and the clinician is again in jeopardy, as well as faced with conflicting agendas. Aided by hindsight, one can always argue about how clear and serious the threat was, whether at least an abbreviated informed consent could have been performed without serious detriment to the patient, and whether the patient was sufficiently "alert and oriented" to appreciate and respond to an informed consent to some extent.

Variations in explicit legal guidance grow out of such variables. Some jurisdictions expand the notion of serious harm to include reversible pain and suffering (Lidz et al., 1984, p. 16). One might also argue that even though disclosure was not immediately possible, a generic consent was possible and should have been solicited. As one source puts it, "it is easy to imagine situations so urgent that full disclosure would be counterproductive but not so urgent that consent, possibly following a highly abbreviated disclosure, could not be obtained" (Appelbaum et al., 1987, p. 69). Further, even in the clear, immediate, and serious situation, one might be faced with a patient who is refusing treatment and exhibits no clear evidence or suggestion of incompetence. Whether the physician honors or ignores such a refusal, either way he seems to face exposure to liability. Ignoring the refusal, however, if the immediate and serious nature of the threat is clear, seems to be the more appropriate measure, both for the patient's own sake and because damages will be awarded only if injury occurs, not just in the absence of informed consent. The law, of course, is appropriately concerned that this exception does not come to undermine the rule. It is unfortunate that its formulation seems to place the well-meaning clinician in jeopardy and leaves him to cope with conflicting agendas.

The Therapeutic Privilege Exception

This exception countenances the withholding of informed consent from a competent patient, as a whole or in part, on the grounds that the informing process itself might directly harm the patient. Various formulations of the nature of the harm at issue exist. At one extreme, we have the traditional concern about the negative psychological effects of giving a patient bad news—for example, that he has a malignant and incurable tumor. At the other extreme we see certain recent legal guidelines that rule out psychological harm as a valid justification and limit this exception only to situations where the harm is immediate and severe, as in an already agitated patient who has unstable angina and inquires about what is happening (Appelbaum et al., 1987, p. 78). Another formulation of this exception keys to competence itself in the sense that "information may be withheld when its disclosure would so upset patients that they would be unable to engage in decision making in a rational way or at all" (Appelbaum et al., 1987, p. 74).

Though we are again faced with an ambiguous and vague rule here, it seems most pertinent to emphasize that the basic issue, in the law as well as the bioethics literature, is whether this exception should be allowed at all. For one thing, the issue of psychological harm has been sharply criticized by the immense discussion of truth telling over the past two decades. The overwhelming, if not unanimous, consensus of this debate is that the likely long-term benefits of truth telling will probably outweigh the short-term conjectured psychological harms (Bok, 1978, pp. 232–55). Equally, even if most of the pertinent information is provided, the absence of a key piece of information (e.g., that the tumor is incurable) impoverishes and corrupts subsequent discussion and experience. As to the concern that the information could "so seriously upset the patient that he could not rationally make a decision," this formulation might be better included in the competency evaluation, as it would not be credible unless there were not already independent grounds for questioning the patient's decision-making capacity. Such an alternative account would not seem to be fully satisfactory in some instances—for example, in a patient with a brittle psychosis who, though presently "alert and oriented," might very likely decompensate if stressful information were provided. But we still do not have a pure case for therapeutic privilege since part of the expected result would be loss of competence. Nondisclosure to such a patient in a situation where the prediction is that he would decompensate but *not* lose competence would be quite controversial. Finally, in instances where probable and severe harm might be postulated (e.g., in the agitated patient with unstable angina), clinicians disagree about whether disclosure could still be offered in a sensitive way without terrifying or devastating the patient *and* thus precipitating a fatal arrhythmia. One could also just as well subsume such situations under the emergency exception with the caveat that once the patient is stabilized, the disclosure must be made.

In sum, though this exception remains on the books in many jurisdictions, it often exists as a quite circumscribed exception and, perhaps, one should look elsewhere to justify any specific nondisclosure.

The Waiver Exception

The least troublesome exception would seem to occur when the patient voluntarily gives up his right to an informed consent. Various reasons may lie behind such an action, including that the patient does not want to be upset by hearing the gory details, or he feels incapable of making decisions and would prefer that his doctor decide. For this exception to be legitimate, the patient should be reminded that he is entitled to such information, and must still give a prior generic consent to treatment, authorizing whatever his doctor believes is best. The issue of whether the waiver is a voluntary one is pivotal here, as when any basic right is waived. Hence, it seems inappropriate for the physician to raise the possibility of a waiver initially, for either all or part of the elements of informed consent, unless the patient has already raised the issue spontaneously.

This exception makes sense in certain situations. The patient who suspects bad news may feel temporarily unprepared to deal with it. It can also, however, conflict with other important agendas—for example, in generating the sort of knowledgeable patient that daily compliance with therapy may well require. It has also been argued that whereas physicians have a duty to disclose information, patients have a corresponding duty to seek to understand it.[15] Further, such a waiver could allow important patient misconceptions and fears to remain unaddressed (or undetected), as well as leave the physician holding the bag of responsibility that the patient should also be shouldering. Finally, there may be personal issues and decisions at hand that are so weighty that there may be no legitimate substitute for the patient's responding to them. As will later be argued, some medical decisions are so fundamentally personal that the physician cannot legitimately offer a recommendation unless the patient speaks specifically to the personal significance of the risks and benefits at hand. We will not, however, be able to become clear about the appropriate scope and place of such waivers until we have a better sense of the goods and values that informed consent might capture and that this particular exception would voluntarily choose not to pursue. Suffice it to say, at this juncture, that we will come to hold that this exception can be particularly troublesome and objectionable in certain cases, and should not be seen as just another way in which a patient exercises self-determination.

SUMMARY

Given that we hope to fashion a model of informed consent that is realistic and effective within clinical medicine, the legal doctrine must be seen as insufficient. Regarding the law's own expressed concern for self-determination, we have seen that it has little positive to say and runs afoul of its own rhetoric to the extent that it tends to motivate clinicians to hyperinform patients "just to be safe." As numerous commentators have pointed out, the law's commitment to self-determination is half-hearted at best (Katz, 1984, pp. 48–84). Further, to the extent that clinicians embrace the law's own focus concerning informed consent, the ritualistic, "damage control" form of informed consent provision tends to be par for the course. If the law tends to treat informed consent primarily as an element within malpractice actions, then it should not be surprised when clinicians respond to the threat and follow its lead. Finally, the law rarely seems to appreciate the basic assaults that illness can make on personal autonomy. It thus offers the clinician a vision of patients as decision makers that appears quite unrealistic, and thus undermines the credibility of its message to those whom it most needs to sway.

We must be careful to be fair to the law here, however. Given that the law's avowed purpose is often to identify what is minimally necessary in our congress with each other, its lack of a full-blown blueprint for this interaction is neither surprising nor lamentable. Surely we do not want to force lawyers to give operationally precise standards for assessing competence or clinical definitions of medical realities, such as what constitutes a medical emergency. They can assist us conceptually, as well as identify practices that fall beyond the pale. But at some point clinical experience and judgment, in concert with the disciplines of bioethics, must speak.

That the law insists on congruence with standards of practice is also fair game and ascertainable by the clinician. Equally, for it to insist that the standard for disclosure must key to what the average reasonable person would tend to find significant rather than simply what clinicians find significant, or feel like talking about, is simply to insist on what the public expects. The law then proceeds by passing on cases where these minimal standards have arguably not been met, thus providing further sense of what it feels obliged to insist upon. Clinically and ethically, we must say that this is not sufficient. But as a matter of what one should expect or hope for from the law, we might well want to thank it for its efforts, and proceed to our wider agenda—namely, what constitutes good clinical practice regarding informed consent. Arguably the law has appropriately restrained itself to only speaking to minimal standards in this regard, not what we might hope for or ethically feel is called for. This more charitable view works only so long as we ignore the background rhetoric of the law (e.g., regarding self-determination) and then go on to note how its malpractice-couched doctrine tends to undermine the pursuit of or provision for such basic principles.

It should also be noted that the medical profession is far from blameless in all of this. For one thing, clinicians who scoff at informed consent as a myth are simply refusing to respond to deeply felt needs of the citizenry. More specifically, the hyperinforming response that certain clinicians have fashioned to combat the risk of suit from nondisclosure is not based on any requirement or recommendation by the law. Suits have been brought and rejected in the case of the nondisclosure of remote risks (Rozovsky, 1984, pp. 66–68). The jeopardy here seems to be quite remote, in fact, and the hyperinforming response thus comes to look more like a hysterical reaction to a very remote threat. We may fault the law for not attempting to reassure the physician who conscientiously tries to follow legal guidance and remains unsure of whether he has actually done so. But we should also fault those clinicians who demand an inordinate degree of reassurance, particularly when we are speaking of a level of risk that clinicians routinely ask patients to face, becoming annoyed with them when they balk. Finally, if the medical profession had voluntarily been more forthcoming and forthright with patients as a matter of its own practice, then the lawyers would not have had cause (or the opportunity) to step in. Clinicians should not have needed lawyers to point out to them the clinical and ethical value of patient understanding, or the fact that some decisions are so value-charged as to go far beyond anything to which professional expertise can univocally speak. If the lawyers have been hyperactive, this was in large part necessitated by the unacceptably hypoactive behavior of clinicians.

The law thus provides us with many questions, doubts, and the grounds for controversy. It calls for debate; it does not resolve it. Further, for those who do not shy away from the use of the law to micromanage behavior (being unable to trust in or appeal to the good will and character of those they want to manage), the law says far too little. However time-consuming the process, such individuals might well seek further legal requirements—for example, that physicians be required not only to disclose information but to ascertain that it has been adequately understood. This requirement could then be supplemented by further ones that require an educational response if the patient's level of understanding is not adequate, as well as counseling and values-clarification responses to the extent special circumstances require them.

So, from one perspective, the law says much less than it should. My clinician reader may feel a bit bewildered, perhaps even outraged, at this point, that anyone would ask for more in addition to the ambiguous, arguably counterproductive doctrine we have just reviewed. Equally, he might suggest, if he still has the patience, that there is little felt or real need in a majority of medical situations for additional hyperinforming and counseling. *It is as if we are to allow an obsession with the extraordinary to dictate our approach to the ordinary.* More fundamentally, common clinical experience seems to raise serious questions about the average patient's capacity to accomplish the cognitive and evaluative tasks involved. In sum, the clinician may well have serious, legitimate doubts about what the lawyer simply presumes without analysis or argument. Given such a discrepancy, it is thus time that we refer to the more fundamental ethical and public policy considerations that generated the doctrine of informed consent in the first place.

NOTES

1. The following is not a history of the legal doctrine of informed consent. At most it identifies major themes in its development. For a detailed history of legal developments regarding informed consent, the reader is directed to *A History and Theory of Informed Consent* by Ruth Faden and Tom Beauchamp, 1986. See also Katz, 1984.

2. The use of the term "self-determination" may be questioned here, as it does not appear in the early cases. I concur with Faden and Beauchamp's argument that this contemporary term best captures the sense of much of the early language of the courts in this regard (Faden and Beauchamp, 1986, pp. 121ff). For example, *Mohr v. Williams*, 95 Minn. 261, 104 N.W. 12 (1905), speaks of the "free citizen's first and greatest right . . . the right to himself" and expresses its concern about "violating without permission the bodily integrity of the patient . . . without his knowledge or consent." The landmark case of *Schloendorff v. Nathanson* 211 N.Y. 128, 105 N.E. 93 (1914), states: "[E]very human being of adult years and sound mind has a right to determine what shall be done with his own body."

3. An early use of the appeal to the right to privacy is found in the *Quinlan* decision, *Quinlan*, 70 N.J. 10, 355 A.2d 647 (1976), a principle later applied in *Roe v. Wade*, 410 U.S. 438 (1972) regarding abortion. See Faden and Beauchamp, 1986, pp. 39ff.

4. See note 2.

5. For a particularly detailed and forceful presentation of this view, see Katz, 1984, pp. 48–84.

6. That informed consents tend to be ineffective has both anecdotal and scientific support, as documented in detail in chapter 3. Their ritual character—monologue statements of risks, benefits, etc.—is a common claim in the literature. Later discussions in this book will repeatedly touch on this "ineffective ritual" issue.

7. It is concurrently worth noting the oft-repeated criticism that this commitment has been half-hearted in that funding to support those transferred out into the community has been meager at best.

8. From the landmark case *Nathanson v. Klein*, 186 Kan. 393, 409 (1960).

9. Established specifically by *Canterbury v. Spence*, 464 F.2d 786, *Cobbs v. Grant* 502 P.2d 1, and *Wilkinson v. Vesey* 295 A.2d 676. See further explanation and citations by Faden and Beauchamp, 1986, pp. 32–33.

10. This third standard bears mention as an option with interesting features. It does not appear to have any formal status in any jurisdiction at present but is often mentioned in accounts of the "doctrine" of informed consent. See commentary and references (especially notes 34 and 36) by Faden and Beauchamp, 1986, pp. 33–34.

11. Since the original edition of this work appeared, a number of attorneys, particularly local colleagues, have challenged me on this. Particularly, a number of them see the tendency in the law to be increasingly away from a professional standard. Anthony Szczygiel, a local attorney-colleague, has extensively "surveyed the informed consent doctrines of the fifty states plus D.C. I found that there is almost an even split on how the disclosure standard is set—twenty-five professional, twenty-two 'reasonable person' or 'subjective patient,' and four others. Counting people rather than jurisdictions, 51 percent of the U.S. population and 53 percent of physicians are in states that have rejected the professional standard of disclosure." He goes on to suggest that "the distinction between the professional and the patient-oriented reasonable person standards is disappearing" (personal communication, June 18, 1996).

I will defer to Mr. Szczygiel here and simply refer the interested reader to his extensive and excellent survey in this regard (Szczygiel, 1994).

12. I discuss whether this is really the law's fault, or an overreaction by clinicians, in my summary remarks at the end of this chapter. In sum, though the law calls for no such hyperinforming, and thus some clinicians *are* overreacting, I feel that the law is equally at fault for not trying to reassure and better inform clinicians regarding the nature and extent of the threat here and how to realistically and efficiently meet it.

13. Technically, the law says to presume competence on the patient's part. It does not ask one to presume that the patient's cognitive and deliberative performance was, in fact, "competently" accomplished. But repeatedly, I submit, the law and lawyers speak as though they also assume that such activities are also occurring in an adequate way.

14. See Rozovsky, 1984, pp. 90–95, for an extended discussion of the elements of the emergency exception.

15. Hull, 1978. See also Morreim, 1991, pp. 133–154.

2

The New Ethos of
Patient Autonomy

Informed consent did not spring full-armored like Athena from the head of Zeus. As already noted, it has undergone a long development in Anglo-American law. Equally, though only in more recent years, the doctrine has been appropriated by a broad-based movement to reform medicine in ways felt to be more congruent with the general practices and aspirations of a free society. And it is to this social movement, this "new ethos of patient autonomy" (McCullough and Wear, 1985; Wear, 1991), that we must now refer in order to understand the ethical agendas, insights, and arguments behind the doctrine of informed consent.

Whether we refer to the law, more popular statements, or the writings of its proponents, the new ethos of patient autonomy comes with certain clear and generally espoused principles and agendas. Given the perception that patients have regularly been as uninformed as they are powerless in health care, the basic prescription has been to inform them and alter that power structure. Impeaching all forms of paternalism, at least for competent patients, the new ethos has advanced the doctrines of informed consent and the right to refuse treatment toward enabling and empowering patients to retain control of their lives in health care. The insistence on truth telling is added to this prescription in recognition of both patients' need for information and insight as to whether there are decisions to be made, and the alleged widespread presence of deception within health care. In sum, in any clinical encounter between competent patients and their health care providers, the essential details of the recommended intervention must be presented to the patient, the patient's consent must be obtained before proceeding, the patient has the right to refuse the intervention without prejudice, and any such interaction must proceed honestly without the presence of lies, deception, or coercion.

29

At some point, however, as the proponents of the new ethos recite their case, one might well wonder how physicians managed to attract any patients at all over the last two millennia. Most people do not appreciate being lied to or deceived, resent being coerced, and supposedly like to retain control of their own lives. In truth, the usual physician-patient interaction was much more benign. Physicians often saw little point in informing patients, preferring to make recommendations that their patients were supposed to accept and with which they were expected to comply. Such behavior may well not have enhanced freedom and self-determination, but neither was it outrageously paternalistic or disrespectful. Both parties in the relationship simply felt that the doctor knew best; such decisions were seen as matters of medical expertise and judgment.

The real impetus for the new ethos of patient autonomy seems to have developed from other, more specific sources and insights, *not*, at least initially, from concern over the silence within the usual physician-patient interaction. Two sorts of clinical situations provided much of the fuel that has made the ethics of medicine such a burning issue in recent years: biomedical research and extraordinary cases.

EARLY CONCERNS ABOUT PATIENT AUTONOMY

Though much is now said about more positive goals of enhancing patient autonomy, the early insights and agendas of the new ethos had a much more negative basis—that medical practice contains profound threats to both patient freedom *and* well-being.

Concerns about Research Subjects

The initial wellspring of such concern was biomedical research. Here, though various demands for informed consent had already been made in response to the specter of the Nazi doctors (Lifton, 1986), it was not until the sixties that this area received the attention it merited. Initially highlighted by members of the medical community itself—for example, in Henry Beecher's article "Ethics and Clinical Research" (Beecher, 1966)—the growing perception was that the biomedical research community had become much too zealous in its dealings with research subjects, who were generally provided little or no informed consent to risky and often nontherapeutic procedures. Further, the populations most often studied were among the most vulnerable and least autonomous in the society. Often research subjects were institutionalized patients, such as prisoners, the mentally ill and developmentally disabled, and the elderly.

Particularly for the medical profession, the problem (and the threat) was clear. Biomedical researchers, in their zeal, had sinned against the traditional principle that the physician's primary allegiance must be to the protection and promotion of the best interests of his patients, regardless of the impact of doing so on other considerations, such as the advancement of medical knowledge. Such physicians were thus coming to the physician-patient relationship with conflicting interests and agendas. In the research setting, the clinician-researcher attempts to benefit not only the patient-subject but future patients as well. That the emphasis had swung intolerably far away from the interests of the research subjects was apparent in numerous instances, such as the Tuskegee and Willowbrook experiments, where, respectively, southern blacks with syphilis were left untreated so that the natural history of the disease could be studied, and developmentally disabled patients were intentionally infected with hepatitis toward the same research goal.[1] Though protests issued from certain quarters, the medical profession itself seemed to recognize the inappropriateness and dangers in such behaviors, and a mandate for informed consent in the research setting gradually evolved, along with the formation of monitoring bodies, or institutional review boards. But such corrections were not accomplished without the growth of a residual distrust within the society that physicians might use patients as guinea pigs.[2]

The Influence of Extraordinary Cases

The new ethos also has deep roots in a consuming focus on extraordinary types of cases. These cases tend to be drawn from the setting of the large, urban, multispecialty hospital, and focus on conflicts between physicians and patients in extraordinary life-threatening situations. Students and teachers of bioethics are familiar with such paradigm cases: adult, competent Jehovah's Witnesses being transfused against their wills; severely burned or spinal-cord-injured patients being sedated or ignored in response to their rejection of aggressive treatment for lives that they do not consider worth living; and adult, competent patients having their lives prolonged in "inhumane" ways, especially in intensive care units, rather than being allowed to "die with dignity," perhaps at home or in a hospice.

We should not miss the images in such cases; they go far beyond mere argument. Whether it be the badly burned Donald Cowart in "Please Let Me Die" (Videotape, 1974), or Richard Dreyfus as a quadriplegic in "Whose Life Is It Anyway?" (Metro-Goldwyn-Mayer, 1981), fuel for moral indignation abounds. In both films, clearly competent and extremely articulate patients are presented as demanding an exit from ghastly and hopeless situations that one might hesitate to wish even on one's worst enemy. And there are the doctors, aloof and arrogant in their white smocks, refusing to honor wishes that any of us might express in such situations, and seeking to circumvent them by drugging their patients, denying their apparent competence, and generally treating them like ignorant, hysterical children.

A REPLY FROM THE PATERNALIST

The preceding images and anecdotes are, however, hardly an appropriate or sufficient basis upon which to generate the across-the-board reformation of modern medicine upon which the new ethos insists. Most patients are not experimental subjects, most health care does not occur in tertiary hospitals or involve life-threatening situations, *and* most patients are not as insightful or articulate as Mr. Cowart or Mr. Dreyfus. Further, it was primarily the medical community itself that corrected the problems in the experimental realm. As to the "please let me die" sorts of cases, I am moved to recall a comment by a senior clinical colleague: "One of my primary duties as a general practitioner was to protect my patients from the specialists."

This last comment suggests an analysis that few proponents of the new ethos seem to have considered—namely, that such therapeutic or experimental zeal was not only *not* common in medical practice but was seen as aberrant by many practitioners. The notion of extraordinary (and thus elective) treatment was around to temper such aggressiveness long before the notion of patient autonomy and the right to refuse treatment had gained currency. The older tradition of beneficence in medicine—paternalism, if you wish—was equally capable of recognizing that there was a point beyond which aggressive maintenance of life provided no benefit and served only to prolong dying and increase suffering. Many senior clinicians have assured me that *this* was the dominant perspective among medical practitioners, *not* the "treat to the bitter end" tendency targeted by the new ethos. As

Hippocrates himself emphasized: "Do not seek to cure patients who are overmastered by disease."

Given that the new ethos does presume to offer a radical reorientation of all medical practice, not just a fine-tuning aimed at certain aberrant behaviors in special circumstances, we will do well here to pause and reflect on the real target of the new ethos, that of medical paternalism. I submit that the controversy is not between the good guys and the bad guys, but rather between two moral visions, each with its own articulate view of what is right and good within health care. Lest our discussion be completely one-sided, as I believe much prior discussion has been, we need to hear from the paternalist.

The reference here is not to the aloof and arrogant technician. The moral vacuum that such an individual creates within the enterprise of caring for the sick is obvious. The real target is, rather, the paternalist who, under the banner of *beneficence* (i.e., commitment to the patients' *best interests*), routinely excludes patients from meaningful participation in decision making. Having had the honor of knowing a few such individuals (one of them, in fact, brought this author, along with his mother and grandmother, into the world), I have always felt that the "doctor-bashing" tenor of certain proponents of the new ethos was inappropriate and destructive. This is so simply because the paternalists' intentions were the noblest and clearly had a substantial factual and ethical base. [3]

The position of the paternalist can be rendered easily enough. Patients come to physicians to be healed (or at least, restored to function and relieved of suffering as much as possible). Given this overriding agenda, the primacy of which both parties agree upon, anything that enhances healing is appropriate, anything that diminishes or undermines it is to be avoided. What enhances it seems quite clear: the *trust* that brings the patient in and generates acceptance, compliance, and cooperation with the physician's recommendations. As to decision making, effective and appropriate management of illness dictates that this is the physician's function. Often there is a clear and primary treatment of choice and the patient comes to the physician to have this identified and provided.

There were other ways to enhance this process as well. Patients also came seeking reassurance, and the physician was loath not to provide it, even if he diverged from or stopped short of the truth. It was, and still is, a common belief among health care professionals that the

more hopeful or optimistic patient does better therapeutically—
responds better *physiologically*—than the more pessimistic, less hopeful patient. If strong reassurance enhances therapeutic response or,
more specifically, if accentuating the positive and downplaying the
negative is therapeutically efficacious, then it would be an abuse of
the patient's trust *and* best interests not to do it.

On this view, truth telling can be countertherapeutic and the
whole new ethos quite misguided. Even now, physicians who are con-
sciously committed to patient autonomy routinely err on the side of
emphasizing the benefits of treatment and the likelihood of success.
The older paternalistic physician simply followed all this to its logical
conclusion. Risks or potential side effects of the treatment were seldom even mentioned, unless they were likely to occur and needed to
be monitored for by the patient himself. Awareness of the placebo
effect, which has been noted to shrink tumors and relieve angina
(Brody, 1982), suggested to the paternalist that the mention of risks
would increase the likelihood that they would occur. Equally, no therapeutic purpose was served by torturing patients with possibilities, or
undermining their confidence by apprising them of the large element
of uncertainty ingredient in most medical assessment and decision
making. Finally, particularly with long and arduous treatments, the
function of the physician was to encourage and stimulate patients'
compliance, rather than allow them to fall prey to their fears or make
tragic choices out of pain, denial, or misconceptions. To do any less
was to fail the patient by not maximizing his chance of recovery. To do
less would equally be to abandon the patient at a particularly vulnerable and crucial hour.

As to patients as decision makers, the paternalist wanted nothing
to do with this, and had no sense that patients wanted anything to do
with it either. How could the average patient, "sick and medically
ignorant" (Rennie, 1980, p. 917), possibly understand, let alone evaluate, the complexities and uncertainties ingredient in a great deal of
medical decision making? And if a case was simple and straightforward, why did the patient need to do so? Did not the patient's presence in the physician's office already indicate that he knew he had a
problem, was not going to just grin and bear it, and had come to have
this problem resolved?

There are, of course, many grounds upon which to quarrel with
the paternalist's argument. Numerous studies, on the one hand, show
that the vast majority of people do want to be informed (Kelley and

Friesen, 1950). *But* other studies have shown that most patients do not think of themselves as the primary decision makers (Alfidi, 1975), and that many prefer that the physician decide in situations of fundamental ethical significance—for example, whether to initiate resuscitative measures in the event of a cardiopulmonary arrest (Wagner, 1985). On the other hand, the doctrine of informed consent does *not* require that patients be tormented with numerous complexities, uncertainties, and possibilities, however remote. Rather, it is the essential risks and benefits that must be provided, the heart of the reasons why the physician decides on one treatment over another. *But* the empirical data and common clinical experience strongly suggest that many patients take little or no interest in informed consent and do not readily embrace the authority and responsibility it seeks to provide (Alfidi, 1975). Finally, endless arguments can be generated in terms of the harms of informing: i.e., whether, to what degree, and how often, revealing the negative side of risks and prognosis is countertherapeutic, specifically by increasing the occurrence of such risks, or by a more general diminishment of therapeutic response.

There is thus much in the preceding sketch of the paternalist's reply about which the defenders of our liberties can wax righteous, even if sick folks somehow neglected to do so over the last few millennia. What we need to hear, however, is not reports of extraordinary cases, or of medical researchers who have forgotten their more fundamental calling, but how, in the main, such beneficence on the part of physicians was inappropriate in the usual case. Thus far we have reason to support informed consent in experimental research and, perhaps, a right to refuse extraordinary treatment. But none of this necessitates a global requirement for informed consent, nor does it give credibility to the notion of patients as decision makers. What we need for the latter theses is an argument that meets the paternalist on his own ground (i.e., beneficence) and speaks to the nature of the typical medical situation. Just such an argument has been offered.

PATIENTS AND PHYSICIANS AS MORAL STRANGERS

In the past, the predominant image was of the wise and beneficent physician, trusted and at times adored by his patients. The new ethos, however, offers us a quite different and rather jaundiced vision. In a nutshell, this view runs as follows. Medicine is an enterprise pursued within a secular, pluralistic society in which physicians and patients meet as *moral strangers* in various senses. First, they are unlikely to *share* the same values and beliefs, given the pluralistic character of medicine and our society wherein people have radically different views of what the good life is and how it is to be pursued and sustained. Second, they are unlikely to *understand* each other's moral views: the patient is, as Engelhardt puts it, "a stranger in a strange land," quite unaware of the special expectations and agendas of his caregivers (Engelhardt, 1986, pp. 256ff). Physicians, for their part, are encased in what Veatch has described as the evolved and idiosyncratic cult of medicine, a cult that remains largely isolated and unresponsive to the culture around it, and gives little status to the patient's perspective within clinical decision making (Veatch, 1972). One still hears physicians declaring that "M.D." means "make decisions." Such a mind-set will not tend to exercise itself overly toward understanding patient values and beliefs. Nor will it tend to be congruent with those values and beliefs, as it still embraces an essentially paternalistic view that is supposedly abhorrent to the citizenry.

Whether or not the preceding is the dominant vision among proponents of the new ethos is not clear. Such an account of the divide between physician and patient clearly enjoys strong support in the writings of such well-known thinkers as Burt, Veatch, Engelhardt, and Katz, the latter two themselves being physicians. My own experience as a teacher of undergraduate medical ethics, among students of diverse backgrounds and avocations, tells me that this vision also captures considerable societal sentiment. Somehow or other, a deep core of distrust has developed regarding the intentions and capabilities of the medical profession.

Such a result should not be all that surprising. However contributory the aforementioned insights regarding medical experimentation and extraordinary cases are, this vision dovetails well with widespread postwar distrust of societal institutions and expertise. Allied to such distrust is the perception that the sciences, biological and otherwise, have been unable to generate sufficient moral sensitivity and insight to match their rapidly expanding knowledge and technical capacity, and that the interests and freedom of the citizenry have been placed in jeopardy as a result.

Equally, this vision, however jaundiced, has an obvious factual base. To be fair, it should be recognized that many health care providers have actively embraced the new ethos. It would simply be erroneous to hold that the average professional is such an arrogant, threatening "other" to his patients. But, however reconstructed, such professionals, along with their patients, are now firmly placed within the assembly-line character of modern medicine. Care and treatment in hospitals are fragmented across loosely coordinated team members and shifts. Often there is either no one clear person directly in charge of the individual patient's care, or even if there is, it is an overworked resident rotating across services, or a tightly scheduled community physician who stops by to check on his patient within a grueling daily marathon from hospital to clinic to private office. Often, in fact, hospitalized patients are essentially doctorless. They are picked up by residents who know nothing of their background and have little or no connection with the patient's private physician (if the patient has one, which he often does not). Further, such residents tend to be quite hesitant even to initiate a personal relationship, or investigate the patient's fears, needs, and desires, as they will probably not have the opportunity to pursue such matters in more than a quite cursory manner. So the personal interaction remains at best pro forma and minimal.

Nor are such problems confined to hospitals or simply the result of the uncaring physician-technician. Anyone presuming to pass judgment on the ills of and silence within modern health care would do well to peruse a recent work concerning the private, rural practice of a young family physician: *Healing the Wounds: A Physician Looks at His Work*, by David Hilfiker (Hilfiker, 1985). In this work we are presented with the specter of a clearly dedicated young doctor, who seems to see the "whole person" quite well. But because of the time constraints and stresses involved, he ends up lamenting his inability to address the underlying psychosocial needs and problems his patients clearly present. Burnout and a flight to a much more anonymous professional situation in a city are the sequelae.

The preceding is bleak but relevant. However well the old country doc may have known his patients, socially and personally, and thus attempted to guide them and make decisions for them, such opportunities have severely atrophied. Clinical medicine is now an enterprise conducted mainly between strangers who do not know each other and may well not share the same values. Thus patient autonomy and informed consent are offered not just as antidotes to arrogant physicians. They are seen as absolute necessities—no one else, in effect, can speak for the patient but the patient.

"This is all very well," our paternalist may reply, "but what leads you to believe that patients are either desirous or capable of stepping into the vacuum here? My common experience is that patients come to me to be fixed and reassured, not educated and forced to make decisions about which they have no expertise. I may know them less well than my forebears, but this has hardly been made up by a corresponding grasp of matters medical by the lay public, particularly given the growth and complexity of medical knowledge. Repeated studies of patient understanding of informed consent have, in fact, shown that the average patient's understanding of even the bare bones of medical situations is abysmal.[4] Further, though I can recognize situations where, given the risks and uncertainties involved, only the patient can truly evaluate them, most medical situations are not so value-charged, none of the patient's basic values are at stake, often a clear recommendation can be made, and that is what the patient expects from me.

"It would be more helpful," the paternalist might continue, "if you were to meet me on my own ground, that of beneficence. In effect, do you have reason to believe that my way of doing things, in fact, is or has been productive of more harm than good? If you could make *that* case, then I would be obliged to change my ways. But so far I feel as if I am watching the evening news where the common experience and perspective of regular people is absent because it doesn't sell Buicks, and we are instead treated to the extraordinary and the bizarre.

"To repeat, I can usually offer a straightforward recommendation to my patients. I also, in varying degrees, advise them about possible outcomes, risks, and complications. If they want more information (few do), I provide it. If they refuse my recommendation, I do not strap them down and force it upon them. I am even willing to admit that certain of the old ways—for example, deceiving terminally ill patients—were misguided and probably often produced more harm than good. But informed consent and patient autonomy still look like farce and delusion to me, and I would like to hear why, at least regarding the issue of who decides, I should see things any differently than I always have. M.D., in fact, does mean "make decisions"; if I cannot do this, my patient is in serious trouble. Or, to quote a fellow traveler, 'if father does not know what is best, he ought to retire from medicine' (Ravitch, 1978, p. 7)."

FREEDOM IN HEALTH CARE

Chapter 4 of this work will respond in detail to the paternalist's specific challenge here, particularly to the beneficence-based issue of what goods and values are lost or slighted by his behavior. The remainder of this work will then pursue a detailed model of informed consent that, realistically and efficiently, attempts to capture these goods and values. But to follow the usual course of argument, the proponent of the new ethos does *not* usually meet the paternalist on his own ground at this juncture. Rather, the autonomist plays his trump card. I pause to consider this "move" *not* because it is telling (I believe it fails), but because it is so common.

The trump card is freedom and it is played roughly as follows. "Let us stop all this quibbling and remember who and where we are. We are members of a free society, and wish such freedom for our fellow citizens as well as ourselves. Thus, whatever the potential harms, and however much patients do not attend to such information, to respond by deleting or downplaying such information removes the very possibility of a person's exercising his freedom of choice. To offer informed consent signals the presence of such choice, and identifies the essential factors on which such choice should be assessed. The patient can still *choose* to embrace, without reflection, the physician's recommendation. Equally, the physician surely retains the option of attempting to persuade the reluctant patient to his view. As to the increase in side effects, or potential diminishment of therapeutic response, such results are clearly not universal, often at most incremental, and seem insufficiently important to justify a blanket policy that would systematically remove freedom of choice from health care. And such a systematic exclusion is simply intolerable.

"Let us remember what it means to be a member of a free society. In our society, all competent people are deemed able and free to manage their own affairs in most areas of human endeavor. With few exceptions, our freedom ensures that we can pursue our lives in terms of our own values, beliefs, and experiences, regardless of how clear or cloudy these are to us, and without concern as to whether others concur with our agendas, or see us as making foolish, stupid, or tragic choices. Moreover, the right to control one's life and the right to be let alone are generally protected from capricious external monitoring as well as circumscription and interference. Competence, as a sociolegal category, is thus *necessarily* seen as a quite low threshold state. One should not have to jump too high a hurdle to attain such status. We should thus presume its presence in adults as the law suggests, and if anyone tends to question it in any particular case, the burden of proof lies with the questioner, a burden that can be satisfied only through the proof of severe mental incapacity or dysfunction. The lawyers have it exactly right."

Practically, then, the reply to the paternalist is that the risks and harms he chooses to emphasize, *even if* we agreed as to their frequency, intensity, and predominance, *must not* be allowed to justify tactics inconsistent with the freedom that we all enjoy in all other areas of human endeavor. Elsewhere, we recognize *and* accept that harm and tragedy may result from the free exercise of one's will. But this is simply the price we must sometimes pay for the freedom to which we give such a fundamental value and status. We thus do not need to meet the paternalist on his own ground—that of beneficence. Even if more harm than good comes of it (however that might be calculated), freedom still trumps.

More theoretically, freedom is not just another value in health care but a regulative principle and a side constraint (Engelhardt, 1982). As long as we are speaking of patients who satisfy the aforementioned low-threshold notion of competence, their freedom *must* be respected. This sense of freedom is simple, straightforward, and negative: one must be free to choose, and given the tendencies of the paternalist, this freedom in health care comes to take the form of *freedom from interference* (McCullough and Wear, 1985), protected and bolstered by informed consent.

It is a central thesis of this work, however, that the preceding does *not* have the force that its proponents take it to have: it is not sufficient to justify the imposition of an across-the-board requirement of informed consent within health care. Further, such argumentation operates under a sense of freedom that is impoverished and merits supplementation.

Freedom from Interference and Informed Consent

Given such a simple and utterly overriding vision of freedom, a vision to which most supposedly assent, one might well wonder why there was ever any question about patient autonomy and informed consent, except from the arrogant, insensitive, or maleficent. It is important, however, not to miss a crucial point about freedom and informed consent in health care: there really is no analogy to informed consent in other areas of human activity. If you want to purchase a new Chevrolet, the salesman is not held to be obliged to ask you if you really want it. Nor is he obliged to refer you to the latest "frequency of repair" data contained in *Consumer Reports*, which would testify to the substantial advantage of certain imports over American-made cars (*Consumer Reports*, 1984, pp. 173–226). Equally, though rather bleak and suggestive of a widespread lack of mutual understanding and compatibility, the statistics regarding divorce are not routinely trotted out as part of the marriage ceremony. In effect, all this talk of freedom certainly mandates the right to refuse treatment. Equally, lies and deception, coercion and manipulation would be ruled out as undermining freedom, as depriving the patient of the chance of even exercising it. But hardly, in any direct way, does any such soliloquy about freedom establish a positive, global requirement for informed consent. Simply, we do not, elsewhere, make knowledge a condition for freedom or generally require a formal declaration of consent. Equally, we do not legally oblige others to inform us, however much we may choose to insist on it in individual cases. We are, as noted, free to proceed, unmonitored, in ignorance, wisdom, or folly, and if we proceed, consent is assumed. Otherwise we would not participate or would walk away. Why, then, is such special treatment required in the clinical setting?

To ask this question is to depart from the practice of many proponents of the new ethos. Generally, the connection between freedom and informed consent is seen as clear and direct. The exercise of freedom requires that the patient consent to the intervention the physician is recommending, and, for this consent to be meaningful, the essentials of what is being recommended must also be provided to the patient. But the point is that generally such a formal process is not required elsewhere in our dealings with one another. Where else are we so fidgety about whether the consent was meaningful? Why, we must ask, are we so concerned to be assured of this in health care?

To ask such questions is, however, to move to the realm where informed consent ceases to be a formality and becomes the vehicle by which numerous agendas and concerns may be addressed. It also involves entering into a realm where numerous barriers to the successful pursuit of such agendas must be recognized. In sum, the suggestion at this juncture is that there are numerous reasons that call for such a special provision. But they go far beyond the concern to maintain freedom from interference in health care.

Restoring Freedom

The primary consideration that mandates informed consent for health care, and not just noninterference, is that freedom is also threatened by what happens to human beings when they are ill. As Edmund Pellegrino has put it, illness often results in "wounded humanity" (Pellegrino, 1979, p. 35). We may be threatened in our very being by such an onslaught. Add to this basic threat other common factors attendant upon illness, such as fear, stress, and confusion, as well as the effects of the pathology (e.g., discomfort and the distraction attendant upon it), and the treatment (e.g., drugs), and the childlike regression often observed in the sick is therefore no surprise (Wear, 1983).

Moreover, particularly in chronic illness, such habitual loss of control would often seem to be the most significant pathological result, meriting as much therapeutic response as bleeding out. And here again, informed consent can be the cutting edge in addressing such regression and the functional loss of freedom it entails. As before, the patient may well opt for reassurance and not decision-making authority, but he has at least been reminded that choices are to be made and risks run. Not that matters are always this simple: the physician may well, at times, feel moved to reject such paternalism-seeking behavior by patients, either as a way to intervene against such regression or simply because the choice at hand is so important, and relative to the particular person's values, that only the patient can speak to it. Informed consent can be instrumental, then, in the attempt to restore the sense of freedom and self-determination so often undermined by illness. Equally, it may also protect such qualities, this time not against the paternalist, but against the patient's own inclinations in a vulnerable and exhausting situation.

In sum, the necessity of informed consent per se throughout health care cannot be based simply on the threat from the medical profession. Though there are interesting exceptions, caveat emptor remains the rule in our dealings with one another. Only with the addition of the sense in which illness undermines human beings in their freedom and self-determination is a move toward such provision necessitated. In this area, freedom is particularly vulnerable and fleeting, and such a unique provision as informed consent may thus be requisite.

The paternalist might well respond to the preceding by pointing out that we have now identified a fundamental ground on which medical paternalism is justified—namely, that sick people are, in fact, undermined in their abilities to control their lives and make decisions. Thus paternalism is the needed response, not the informed consent ritual. The abilities to understand, evaluate, and make choices are all diminished by factors commonly present in illness, such as fear, stress, pain, confusion, and denial, and these are the very abilities needed in informed consent.

Enhancing Freedom

The advocate of the new ethos may respond, in turn, that while such diminishing factors may well be legion, they usually do not *obliterate* competence, which is, as noted, a low-threshold notion. Their presence, rather, instructs us that the ability to be self-determining is at risk to the onslaught of illness. Thus special tactics, such as informed consent and a general concern to protect and restore autonomy, are needed. And the trump card here, the autonomist will insist, remains freedom. There is only one way to respond to such factors: seek to remove or mitigate them in individuals who still retain the necessary conditions for the free exercise of their wills.

The enterprise of enhancing freedom, in fact, may well be of greater import than any of the preceding. The situation of illness does involve threats to freedom. Equally, and at times primarily, it calls for the special expression and exercise of it, and informed consent can be an important management tool in this regard as well.

By way of example, consider the silent killer, borderline hypertension. What is involved in its treatment? Perhaps most essentially, it is the project of persuading asymptomatic patients to take antihypertensive medications that will make them feel worse, and chronically so, than they felt prior to diagnosis. Allied to this, significant tasks of compliance, cooperation, and self-monitoring must be performed by such patients. One should wonder what more crucial and potentially effective intervention the physician can perform in such situations than a full informed consent to encourage such behavior, particularly in people who usually have not been chronically ill before and are used to taking their bodies and health for granted. Any technician can diagnose and prescribe for hypertension. It takes a skilled clinician to stimulate the enhanced exercise of self-determination needed to meet such a situation. In such a case, the basic tool for medical management is informed consent.

A second important way in which informed consent can enhance freedom appears if we move away from worrying about how to protect it in its most minimal sense and reflect on the more positive reasons why we value freedom in the first place. We value freedom because we much prefer to weigh these choices and options

ourselves, *in terms of our own personal values, beliefs, and life experiences.*
Clinical medicine is just such an arena of choices. As recent work in
clinical decision analysis illustrates, the evaluation of *any* treatment
involves a more or less explicit, integral consideration of the probability of occurrence multiplied by the value or disvalue of the risks and
benefits of the procedure (Weinstein et al., 1980). In other words,
every clinical decision involves value judgments regarding risks to be
run for benefits sought and the payoff or price of pursuing one treatment over another or over no treatment at all. Given such choices, a
more positive sense of freedom suggests that informed consent can be
used as the basic medium within which the physician assists the
patient to recognize and evaluate such choices in terms of the
patient's unique values, beliefs, and life experiences. We thus should
recognize a broader enterprise of values clarification and negotiation,
and the tailoring of medical management to it. Informed consent thus
receives its marching orders, in part, from the enterprise of enhancing freedom.

The practicing clinician might well object that aside from there
being only so many hours in the day to accomplish such "counseling," there often is no need for it. The patient's basic values and beliefs
are often *not* at stake and the choice is clear. The patient who comes to
the physician with pneumonia, and for which ampicillin is the treatment of choice, hardly needs to accomplish some broad existential
reflection. At most he needs to be encouraged to take the pills and be
advised as to why he should take all of them and not just stop when
he feels better. In sum, we may well have added credibility to
informed consent and communication in the situation of chronic illness here, but even this, along with experimentation and extraordinary cases, still speaks to the minority of medical cases. We may have
gotten in some good licks on the periphery of medicine, but still a global prescription for informed consent, especially in the common area
of ordinary, everyday treatment, is not justified by the facts of the matter or patients' interests.

The Heterogeneity of Clinical Needs and Tasks

Response to this objection leads us to a final conviction about
informed consent that will come to be a basic touchstone of the argument of this work. This conviction is not only that the negative "freedom from interference" view is impoverished both in terms of the
meaning of freedom and with regard to what informed consent can

accomplish. More basically, such a view, both theoretically and in practice, assumes a homogeneity of needs and tasks within clinical decision making that is simply not the case. We should agree that values clarification and counseling are not needed in the prescription of ampicillin for pneumonia. Such counseling is, in fact, probably not needed in much of medicine where the clinician is comfortable with a given recommendation and the patient willingly consents to it. *At least on the score of protecting, enhancing, or restoring freedom, there is often no significant call for a detailed informed consent or an allied counseling response.*

By contrast, what of the patient with newly diagnosed metastatic disease or an evolving chronic condition? *Substantial* value choices arise in such situations, and the patient may well need much time, reflection, and counseling to respond to them. And we should probably speak of *establishing* rather than simply *identifying* the patient's views regarding such situations. We can hardly expect patients' views to be adequately worked out regarding unanticipated and extraordinary scenarios. The negative "freedom from interference" view of freedom and informed consent recognizes no such further needs and tasks. Rather, it absurdly frets about protecting patients from those who may well be their only source of insight and support. Informed consent then is advocated univocally for all clinical situations without regard for the heterogeneity of needs and realities that exists across the spectrum of clinical medicine. Further, by being reticent to recognize the diminishments and vulnerabilities often attendant upon illness, the "freedom from interference" view fails to recognize two corollary realities: (1) that patients often need help and encouragement toward accomplishing further reflection and insight and (2) that sometimes they are essentially incapable of doing so.

Finally, beyond such values clarification and negotiation, other important needs, crucial to freedom and self-determination, also arise in certain clinical situations. In evolving chronic illness, patients need to go far beyond simple treatment decisions. Often their lives are going to be inescapably affected in profound ways that they must come to appreciate and to which they must adapt. They may need to be assisted to anticipate further developments of their clinical course so they can rearrange their activities as well as their aspirations and plans. They may need to fashion an interpretation for themselves of what it means to live with a handicapping condition or an ongoing threat to life. In sum, the patient must make judgments about what kind of person he has become now that he is chronically ill or seriously threatened. Clearly the physician is an essential resource within such an enterprise. And informed consent needs to be part and parcel of it.

THIS IS ALL VERY WELL AND GOOD, BUT . . .

My clinician reader may find the preceding more palatable than the usual soliloquy on informed consent and patient autonomy, but enthusiasm for the project may not have been generated. One might agree that the paternalist, given the contemporary assembly-line character of medicine, has lost the essential ground of his presumption—that of an intimate knowledge of the patient for whom he presumes to decide. Such agreement might then lead to the enshrinement of a right to refuse treatment and truth telling so that the patient, as a stranger in a strange land, at least has a veto that must be addressed. The force of a physician's authority with most patients is not necessarily diminished thereby, and the option of persuasion is still available when needed. Equally, some sense of the precarious nature of patient autonomy has been recognized, so at least the usual delusions about patients' abilities to understand and make decisions are not being repeated.

But we are still a long way from the conclusion that every patient needs and will truly profit from an informed consent. Though freedom and patient autonomy demand truth telling and the right to refuse treatment, they do not necessarily require the across-the-board provision of informed consent. Further, one will hopefully agree that chronically or terminally ill patients, as well as those facing major, risky interventions, need to understand their situation and prospects, not just for the purpose of making decisions, but to appreciate and adapt to threatened or actual changes in their life circumstances. But the last caveat speaks to a small segment of medical care. In most clinical encounters the situation is, in fact, as noted: a patient has come to a physician to be fixed and reassured, and the physician is ready, willing, and able to make a clear recommendation as to how this might be accomplished. Or, as the physician Eric Cassell has put it, often the best way for the clinician to protect or restore patients' autonomy is simply to cure them (Cassell, 1977). Why then retain a global requirement for informed consent? Are we not thus back to an activity whose ineffectiveness is well documented by empirical studies?[5] And are we not just wasting precious time, time that might better be spent on other agendas rather than on a ritual that neither physicians nor most patients see any need for? If either do see such a need in a specific instance, they will provide or request it. But why require it when neither spontaneously pursues it?

RETROSPECT AND PROSPECT

Pausing to take stock at this juncture, it seems fair to say that our dialectic has advanced beyond a simple confrontation between the autonomist and paternalist perspectives. Clearly the traditional paternalist perspective per se cannot be sustained as it offends against basic societal values regarding the protection and enhancement of freedom. But, concurrently, we should note that the view that sees patient autonomy and informed consent as a panacea for the "silence" within medicine fares no better. This silence, on the one hand, may often not be objectionable in many instances. On the other hand, the requisite response to this silence in certain particularly poignant situations may have to go far beyond anything the proponents of the new ethos have envisioned. Many of the previously expressed needs and goals are only occasionally and in degree at stake in the clinical encounter, and significant skepticism is in order regarding how effectively they can be met.

We thus end this chapter inconclusively and with the essential confrontation intact. Nor is there any clear and simple resolution available. The autonomist would clearly enjoy the sanction and support of the lay public regarding the goals *and* presumptions previously noted—for example, the presumption of competence and the goal of generating informed patients. But the skeptical clinician still enjoys the authority of experience and can legitimately continue to maintain that such goals and agendas clash with the actual needs and opportunities ingredient in clinical medicine. Even a cursory look at the literature in this area shows repeated volleys across the no man's land that separates the two perspectives, advancing the debate not one bit.

We are thus faced with a situation of thesis and antithesis, of two partial and flawed but nevertheless insightful perspectives, which must somehow be synthesized. That such a synthesis is neither obvious nor readily available is one point of this chapter. That a synthesis, or at least some agreed-upon common ground, has not emerged after so much debate in the literature signals that we will have to dig deeper to find it, and we must somehow do justice to both sides in the process. The next chapter, on "The Clinical Experience of Patient Autonomy and Informed Consent," will pursue some of this necessary excavation.

NOTES

1. Beecher, 1966.

2. Arthur Caplan, in his review of the first edition of this book, asserts that I gave less significance than is merited to the role of biomedical research in advancing the doctrine of informed consent. Perhaps; but he certainly gives more content to this area than I have in this section, and I commend his review to the reader for further detail (Caplan, 1995).

3. There are various sources of paternalism in medicine, some credible, some not. I am concerned here with the variety that bases its actions on an articulate vision of patients' best interests and the threats to these interests in the situation of illness. Paternalism can also spring from a penchant for convenience and control, at times ego gratification and arrogance, that proceeds by ignoring the needs and concerns of patients, as well as the value-charged character of medical decision making. The latter sources of paternalism, I submit, are simply pathological in clinicians, have no credence, and merit no response other than contempt and sanction.

4. See chapter 3 for extensive discussion in this regard.

5. See chapter 3 regarding such ineffectiveness.

3

The Clinical Experience of Patient Autonomy and Informed Consent

Any attempt to characterize the dominant view of clinicians on patient autonomy and informed consent is precarious at best. On the one hand, the new ethos of patient autonomy is hardly just an outsider's fabrication, fashioned by lawyers and philosophers. Indeed, some of its most forceful and well-known advocates have been physicians—for example, Howard Brody, Eric Cassell, H. Tristram Engelhardt, Jr., Jay Katz, and Edmund Pellegrino. On the other hand, the clinical literature is replete with heartfelt attacks on the "myth of informed consent" (Ravitch, 1978), a view often echoed on the firing line.

But we are not really faced with a choice between complete rejection or affirmation. Clinicians will hopefully accept the idea that some laypersons can grasp much of the essence of the choices facing them, and some patients evolve sophisticated appreciations of their situations and prospects. Equally, the value of patient understanding for compliance, cooperation, and self-monitoring is apparent. Finally, extensive and repeated discussions are needed to enlist and maintain chronically or terminally ill patients in extended or extraordinary treatment regimens. The possibility that extraordinary treatment may result in no more than extra suffering without cure is increasingly well recognized in many families from the prior experience of a loved one. The resultant fear and reticence may require a substantial informational and counseling response.

But if we go beyond admissions that some patients are quite capable of autonomous decision making, and that patient understanding is often desirable as well as necessary, the prevailing view of clinicians still seems to involve a rejection of the most basic and revolutionary presumption underlying the new ethos and informed consent— namely, that most patients are sufficiently capable of understanding, evaluating, *and* making decisions about their medical situation and prospects. In part this negative view is grounded in well-known clinical studies that are seen as severely questioning the assumptions of the new ethos and the efficacy of informed consent. But, more basically, many physicians simply feel that the basic assumptions of the new ethos do not square with the day-to-day realities of clinical medicine. What are the root causes of this skepticism?

CLINICIAN PERSPECTIVES ON PATIENT AUTONOMY AND INFORMED CONSENT

Distilled from a host of conversations with my clinical colleagues over two decades, the prevailing clinician perspective on patient autonomy and informed consent would seem to be this: most patients come to physicians for their expertise in identifying and resolving problems that the patient no longer wants to grin and bear. In short, they come to be fixed and, to the extent necessary, reassured. They usually do *not* come to be educated, often not even listening to whatever information is provided, and do not see themselves as decision makers regarding matters about which they have no expertise and of which they are often quite ignorant. Further, patients are prudent in this regard since they often have as many misconceptions about their problems as they do insights. For them, the "essence" of the decision at hand is often just a quite abstract snapshot of a much more complex, uncertain, and evolving situation. Finally, even if patients are interested in and capable of understanding their situation and prospects, there is seldom time for them to internalize and deliberate about such matters, at least in a fashion that would make their consent other than knee-jerk and unreflective. Informed consent is thus a fiction masking a much simpler reality—that of the patient who chooses whether or not to *trust* in his physician's judgment. In sum, patient autonomy and informed consent may be, at best, "fast ethics," as in "fast food," and one may well wonder about the amount and quality of the "beef" inside the roll. And, for clinicians, the preceding is endlessly reconfirmed in their practice day in and day out. Whatever the new ethos is offering, it is *not* a description of the spontaneous behavior of patients or a report of what they tend to request or pursue when faced with significant illness.

Hand in hand with such experience of patient autonomy and participation in medical decision making stands the traditional clinician commitment to the patient's well-being—the much maligned principle of beneficence. Not only is the usual patient seen as insufficiently capable of real decision making, but various unnecessary harms may redound to the patient to the extent this is pursued. The insistence that risks and complications be mentioned to patients creates a negative placebo problem (a nocebo, if you will); that is, if a certain possible side effect of a drug is mentioned, the likelihood that that side effect will occur is increased. Remember that there is almost always a physiological response to placebo in controlled studies, and that it has been thought, somehow, to shrink tumors and relieve angina pain (Brody, 1980). A pertinent example is a drug that occasionally causes impotence. Given the psychological dimension of impotence in many cases, anyone in the least concerned about the patient's well-being might well wonder if it is really necessary to mention such a side effect, particularly since, if impotence occurs, removal of the drug will not necessarily remove its sequelae. For such reasons, in fact, certain clinicians have wondered whether informed consent not only is a myth but might also be "harmful to one's health" (Fries and Loftus, 1979). Beyond this nocebo problem, clinicians are also concerned that informed (but uneducated and frightened) patients might make foolish, stupid, or tragic choices, particularly by refusing appropriate treatment, and many clinicians seem to have a poignant anecdote of just such an occurrence. That such disasters do not routinely occur may comfort the proponent of patient autonomy, but this lack of wholesale harm is not going to impress the clinician who does not see the point of such autonomy in the first place.

By way of qualification, I do not have the sense that the previous sentiments indicate that a rabid paternalist lurks in most physicians. Most seem committed to advising patients about their essential problems and prospects. Equally, few seem to relish the enterprise of forcing treatment on a patient who is refusing it. Rather, the consensus would simply seem to be that, although truth telling is appropriate and the competent patient's refusal of treatment should be honored, it is the process of informed consent, and the presumptions behind it, that do not bear analysis. Such informing has its own harms and risks them in pursuit of a will-o'-the-wisp that is usually not sought, desired, or attainable by the average patient—that is, autonomous and knowledgeable patient decision making. If the patient insists on more information, it should be provided. If he refuses treatment, generally that refusal should be honored, however grudgingly, and with an appropriate counseling response.[1] But, please, let us not waste precious time pursuing the undesired, unattainable, and, quite possibly, harmful.

EMPIRICAL STUDIES OF INFORMED CONSENT

There is strong, albeit ambiguous, support for much of the preceding "clinical perspective" from the many empirical studies of informed consent. Numerous studies have found that the average patient can, at best, identify only half of the information supplied. Other studies show much lower levels of understanding.[2] All of these studies have significant design flaws, which we must also review, but certain findings occur repeatedly and merit identification and evaluation.

Patient Understanding of Disclosed Information

There are numerous studies of the general effectiveness of informed consent that measure the percentage of patient recall of the total information provided. Their results vary markedly, but none show a particularly rosy picture. The best results were obtained by Bengler et al., who found that 72 percent of disclosed information was retained immediately after provision (Bengler et al., 1980). This percentage, not surprisingly, dropped to 61 percent at three months post disclosure. At the other extreme, Robinson and Merav found only 20 percent recall of information at four to six months post disclosure (Robinson and Merav, 1976). The bulk of the studies show recall rates within the 30 to 50 percent range.[3]

There are good reasons to quarrel about the significance of all such studies, depending on one's bias. The four-to-six-month lag time of the Robinson study probably means that it is the result of the natural forgetting process over time that is being documented. This study's 20 percent recall rate hardly proves that patient understanding, *at the point of consent*, was that low. Many of the studies were, in fact, conducted well beyond the point of consent and treatment, and thus erroneously tend to conflate remembering with understanding. Others contain no sense of what was actually said to patients, or how it was presented. In short, such studies offer no sense or reassurance regarding the content and quality of the communication the study subjects received. One study, however, by Morgan and Schwab regarding cataract lens replacement surgery (Morgan and Schwab, 1986), seems to escape such flaws by providing a relatively simple informed consent and a test of patient understanding on the day after surgery. This study found a 37 percent rate of overall understanding. Risking ageism, one might argue, however, that its one design flaw lies in the fact that its average patient age was seventy-five, with no attempt to identify incompetent patients, or note that perhaps this result is a function of a population that is particularly prone to "let doctor decide," as this is what the elderly are used to.

Additionally, no study has documented an overall understanding rate of over 72 percent, and the average of all of them would probably be around 50 percent. This, at least, indicates that optimism about the effectiveness of informed consent is not warranted, at least in the sense of information acquisition. Further, those studies that tested for specific elements of informed consent reported particularly troublesome findings. In Morgan's study, even if one worries about the number of unidentified incompetents in his elderly population, only 4 percent of the patients recalled more than two of five disclosed risks, the most alarming risk of blindness was recalled only by one-third, and 95 percent did not remember three out of the five mentioned complications. Finally, only 50 percent remembered either of the two alternative treatments, and 16 percent could not even recall that they were given an informed consent (Morgan and Schwab, 1986, p. 42).

Now the preceding low levels of recall, and the absence of any study showing high recall of even the "essentials," question any optimistic view of informed consent. Morgan and Schwab, for their part, concluded that the poor results called for an "excessive pursuit of informed consent," but they did not indicate what such an "excessive pursuit" would involve or why, given their relatively simple and straightforward approach, a more intensive pursuit would be more effective (Morgan and Schwab, 1986, p. 45).

Other Empirical Findings

Aside from the comprehension of information, numerous other empirical findings seem to confirm the anecdotal views of clinicians that we previously identified. Cassileth et al. found that understanding decreased as the degree of illness increased, an expected result that common clinical experience supports (Cassileth et al., 1980). A number of studies showed that patients do not seem to take the informed consent process seriously,[4] a majority not even reading the consent forms carefully, and that "most believed consent forms were meant to protect the physician" (Cassileth et al., 1980, p. 896; President's Commission, 1983, p. 108). Others found that patient understanding was quite idiosyncratic and related more to the patient's own past experience than to the information the physician provided (Fellner and Marshall, 1970; Faden and Beauchamp, 1980). And a couple of studies documented some degree of "nocebo" effect in that certain side effects seemed to increase in intensity and occurrence as a result of disclosure (Cassileth et al., 1980, p. 896; Loftus and Fries, 1979; Cairns, 1985).

On the other side of the ledger, however, certain empirical findings contradicted common clinician views. Consistently, studies have found that most patients (usually above 90 percent) definitely wanted to be informed and participate in the decision making (Alfidi, 1971), and that physicians routinely underestimated such patient desires (Faden and Beauchamp, 1980). Such opinions were often gained from healthy people or stable patients, who may well, as clinicians often suggest, not be so interested when they are sick and in jeopardy, but the latter tendency has not been empirically substantiated.[5] Further, the concern that informing patients will lead to an increase in the refusal of treatment has been generally disproved. In fact, not only has such an increase not occurred, but it has been found instead that treatment refusals tend to increase when patients are *not* informed (Faden and Faden, 1978; Leydhecker et al., 1980; Morgan and Schwab, 1986). Finally, numerous studies have documented a significant discrepancy between what physicians think their patients want and what those patients actually do desire (Bedell and Delbanco, 1984, p. 1089; Uhlmann et al., 1988, p. 115).

The problem of increasing anxiety, particularly by mentioning the risks of treatment, has also been extensively studied. While a few studies report that anxiety was increased to some extent (Leeb et al., 1976), most seem to indicate that anxiety is not increased and often is reduced when patients are better informed (Freeman et al., 1981; Morgan and Schwab, 1986). There is also substantial evidence that informed consent is a key factor in patient satisfaction and that informed patients cope with and adapt to situations better (Cassileth et al., 1980; Wallace, 1986). It has also been shown that anticipating the occurrence of pain tends to decrease its felt intensity, while more anesthesia is needed in the absence of such an anticipation (Wallace, 1986, p. 32). Finally, to the common criticism that informed consent takes too much time, one study found that clinicians overestimated the time spent giving informed consent by a factor of 9 (Waitzkin and Stoeckle, 1976).

Implications of These Findings

These studies, with their flaws, conflicting findings, and differing contexts, yield something for everyone. Proponents of informed consent can point to enhanced coping and adaptation to situations, the reduction of pain and anxiety, and a higher rate of acceptance of treatment. Further, however short of perfect recall, proponents can call for enhancing the process *and* insist that some degree of understanding is better than none at all.

On the other hand, those who oppose (or are at least lukewarm about) informed consent retain the option of insisting that its effectiveness is shown to be, at best, marginal by the preceding data. They can continue to hold that informed patient participation in decision making is not an outcome that one should assume is easily gained or merits striving for. The law's unqualified presumption of patient competence is thus clinically impeached. In effect, clinicians may still be justified in believing it foolish to approach the average patient as a capable co-participant in decision making. Further, whatever the suggestions from the enthusiasts, there is no evidence that an "excessive pursuit" of informed consent will result in any significant increase in patient understanding. Finally, we must note that such results regarding patient understanding relate only to the bits and pieces of informed consent. Even a strong showing in this regard hardly reassures us that patients will be able to move to the more complex and difficult stage of evaluation and deliberation regarding such "bits and pieces" with a similar level of success.

Our own conclusion must be that neither side wins the day thus far. However much the proponents of informed consent have societal support and the weight of rhetoric on their side, their enterprise surely remains marginal when it comes to actual effectiveness. One earlier comprehensive evaluation of these empirical studies, in fact, concluded that "whether informed consent is or is not feasible is still an open question" (Roth and Meisel, 1981, p. 2476). Fifteen years of studies later, we must still entertain the same conclusion. Though certain benefits, such as enhanced compliance, coping, and a diminished experience of anxiety and anticipated pain, seem to clearly derive from informed consent, the informed patient as decision maker has just not materialized. And to pursue the former does not require belief in the latter.

The converse conclusion that informed consent is a myth is no more tenable. There is no reason to assume that competent persons attain substantially higher levels of insight in any other area of activity than the preceding groups of subjects. The empirical studies of informed consent may simply be reporting the level of understanding people bring to all of their endeavors. But we are hardly going to conclude from this that freedom is a bad idea and turn the management of our lives over to experts. Equally, opponents of informed consent are placed in the tenuous position of quarreling with strong patient preferences, basic societal presumptions, and the agendas of society's elected representatives (i.e., as seen in informed consent statutes and court findings), to the extent they wish to reject the process of informed consent as not *sufficiently* effective to such agendas. Such a radical conclusion clearly bears the burden of proof in a free society; at least in this sense, freedom does trump.

The preceding does not, however, constitute the sort of adequate investigation of the clinical experience of patient autonomy that we can and should perform at this juncture. Even if clinicians' views are often anecdotal, and the results of empirical studies ambiguous, much more needs to be said about certain relevant clinical realities. We should recall Pellegrino's contention that sickness results in "wounded humanity." This effect of illness creates a need for informed consent as well as allied counseling responses, but it equally raises questions about the actual abilities of the "wounded" to make decisions.

DIMINISHED COMPETENCE

We have noted that the law presumes that the adult patient is competent to participate in decision making and give informed consent. In one sense, such a presumption serves the important goal of protecting patients' legal status as free citizens who retain control over their bodies and their affairs. This presumption also tends to sustain such status in gray areas—that is, when the patient's actual cognitive and decision-making capacities are marginal. This is arguably appropriate. Even if the patient lacks a detailed sense of his situation and prospects, he may still be sufficiently in touch with his basic values and life experiences to assess whether the proposed intervention is congruent with them. The low-recall studies are disconcerting; they are not damning. They do, however, surely undercut any facile optimism about patient decision making, and any such optimism completely evaporates once one attends to the realities of illness and health care, as we shall now do.

As citizens and potential patients, we would tend to subscribe to the preceding, but as clinicians it can be quite troubling. Many factors that clearly tend to diminish patients' abilities to understand, evaluate, and decide are often present in a given patient. Whether such factors actually place the patient below the threshold of competence is an issue that we will return to later in fashioning an operational notion of competence (see chapter 7). For now, our task is simply to identify those factors and reflect upon their potential effect on patients' decision-making abilities. We can certainly quarrel about the degree to which such abilities are to be required, or the significance of any such diminishing factor, especially regarding a summary judgment of whether a given patient is competent or not. It seems undeniable, however, that such diminishing factors are both often present and numerous, thus advising us that the competence the law asks us to presume, or the abilities we hope for, may only be marginally present.

Finally, many of these diminishing factors are commonly present and, alarmingly, often increase in intensity and number as the health of the patient decreases. In other words, competence tends to become questionable in exactly those situations when it is particularly important for patients to understand and participate in decision making.

Before we address such issues, however, we must first identify the diminishing factors involved. Fear, stress, and anxiety are common and surely can diminish a patient's mental abilities, as can pain, drugs, and the confusion often attendant upon illness. Many other sorts of diminishing factors can also be identified.

Factors Ingredient in Illness

Metabolic abnormalities, or poor oxygenation of the brain from pulmonary or vascular deficits, have mental sequelae, as is the case with physical discomfort, clinical depression, and lethargy. Numerous anecdotes exist of patients with such deficits who, while satisfying minimal competency requirements, refused treatment, but later did not even remember they had said anything of the sort and were glad to have somehow survived. Equally, certain comorbidities of severe illness (e.g., uremia in renal insufficiency or hypercalcemia in advanced carcinoma) definitely tend to obtund patients who may still, on the surface, seem to be alert, oriented, and able to respond appropriately. Particularly when we think of the "essay mode" of decision making, which is surely what we hope patients would attain in decision making, such surface presentations are not reassuring.

Common Psychological Responses to Illness

The passive nature of the sick role has long been recognized (Peabody, 1927), particularly in the way it often tends to produce an almost childlike state of regression. Such a traditional description may not be value-neutral since paternalistic physicians may have tended to see what their ideology leads them to expect. Equally, paternalistic behavior—Jay Katz's "silence" at the bedside—may well have been as much a cause of as a response to such regression. Any reflection on what actually happens to patients as they enter the health care milieu (e.g., waiting helplessly until seen, being asked to remove their clothes, etc.) can also be seen as contributory. It at least seems accurate to say that patients have traditionally been given little opportunity, encouragement, or assistance to be other than passive, and much routinely occurs that would tend to both shore up and produce such passivity.

But such regression in patients is too common and significant to attribute it solely to clinician behavior or the nature of health care delivery. The previously mentioned needs to be fixed and reassured are clearly not autonomy-enhancing factors, however common and "normal" such responses to the threat of illness are. Such a passive orientation can also clearly result in patients not listening to or being interested in the tasks of informed consent, as well as being overly submissive to or respectful of physician expertise. At times such passive behavior appears similar to the behavior of an animal that freezes when faced with or grasped by a predator. Denial, for its part, may well be adaptive and appropriate (or, at least, "normal") at certain junctures, but it remains, by definition, a refusal or inability to recognize the facts of one's situation and prospects (a necessary condition, one would think, of informed consent and competence). Denial might thus be seen as just such a freezing in a cognitive sense, as might other passive behaviors commonly witnessed in patients—for example, not reading the consent forms, or not asking the doctor questions that one has (commonly reported by nurses). Finally, patients may trust physicians too much or too little, may appear extremely hospital- or risk-averse, and may well be keying to past experiences of their own, or of loved ones, that are not analogous to their present situations. One poignant personal example of this was a woman who presented with an eminently resectable, discrete bowel tumor and who, on having received confirmation that she had cancer, concluded that she was in the same situation as her sister who had recently died of an untreatable pancreatic carcinoma. She steadfastly refused counseling and treatment.

Long-Term Psychological Characteristics

The etiology of patient passivity is thus multifactorial, not just iatrogenic, and no modification of clinician behavior or health care delivery is likely to remove it completely. It appears to be a relatively normal response to illness. Moreover, for many patients, it may just be their standard way of dealing with life, not just illness. Many people, in varying degrees, are basically passive and have no urge or habit of decision making, having been more directed than autonomous in their work situations as well as their family units. Often such individuals, when asked what they wish to do, will throw the ball back immediately, either at the physician or at a dominant family member. Equally, some come with unrealistically optimistic or pessimistic views about treatment, or life itself, which, to the onlooker, may be more suggestive of a personality disorder than anything one would tend to see as autonomously held views.

There are also many patients who, even though they might pass a mini-mental status exam, are ill and in the hospital as a direct result of self-destructive behaviors. Obesity, alcoholism, smoking, and drug addiction are often the primary etiology of many patients' ills and if patient autonomy means anything, one should assume that they are aware of the effects of such behaviors. Often they are. And one is then left wondering whether and in what sense the core meaning of autonomy, being self-determining, can be meaningfully present in such patients. Once again, satisfactory completion of a mental status exam is hardly going to be very reassuring.

Other Diminishing Factors

The patient with little education, a short attention span, an impaired memory, a past stroke, or a history of mental illness hardly inspires confidence, nor do those who simply do not seem very bright. Patients may come with needs that conflict with autonomy, like the patient who tries to solicit reassurance beyond what the facts of his case afford. Attention-seeking or manipulative behavior can be manifested in refusals of treatment as well as noncompliance. Some patients are clearly being manipulated by family members with their own rather bizarre or conflicting agendas. Equally, a patient may find that he has been abandoned by family and supposed friends precisely at the point when such support systems are most needed. How much easier, then, is it for such people to give way to the counsel of their fears? Or, as an old saying puts it, "A man alone is in bad company."

The preceding excursion should provide substantial credence to the clinical skepticism about decision-making competence in the sick. Such factors are not that rare and are often conjointly present in patients. We may well ultimately stay with the law's presumption of competence, however much realism dictates that we should often add the word "diminished" to it. Beyond realism, it also seems fair to say that however minimal our requirements for the status of competence are, it is often going to fall short of what we would certainly hope for and, particularly when the decisions at hand are poignant, be the cause of true alarm. Whether and to what extent the law and society should maintain their low threshold presumption about competence will be reviewed later. That many patients are not as bright-eyed and bushy-tailed as we might hope is surely also the case; nor is this all.

EXTERNAL BARRIERS TO
PATIENT AUTONOMY AND INFORMED CONSENT

Numerous other clinical factors tend to serve as barriers to patient competence, however intrinsically robust or marginal it is. Some of these factors stem from the nature and environment of contemporary health care; others are intrinsic to the character of the decisions that clinicians and patients face.

Institutional Barriers

Contemporary health care is provided in a milieu that is at least not autonomy-enhancing and may often have a quite diminishing influence as well. Care is usually provided by strangers who are unlikely to know the patient personally in any meaningful way, nor will time usually be available to rectify this. Alienation is thus a built-in feature of the health care assembly line. It seems safe to assume, in fact, that a given patient's caregivers do not share that patient's basic values and beliefs. This seems apparent when one reflects on the sorts of people who become physicians. They are a breed apart. The drive and ambition, the willingness to accept a long and, at times, brutal apprenticeship for the sake of a distant goal, the bias toward life and belief in the power of technology and science—these are all exceptional beliefs and behaviors, not the rule. There may equally be a linguistic or cultural mismatch between the patient and physician where one's meaning or implication is completely lost on or fundamentally misconstrued by the other.

The lack of time is a crucial factor. Not only does it usually preclude the growth of an in-depth relationship between physician and patient, but it has other detrimental effects. All communication or counseling between the parties, including informed consent, must be sandwiched in between many other diagnostic and therapeutic agendas. This tends to dictate that the former activities will at best be discrete, circumscribed events. They will not occur in an unfolding process of mutual exploration, feedback, and understanding that we might hope for, the sort of intervention that might truly be expected to produce patient understanding.

In effect, contemporary health care has taken on many of the features of an assembly line, none of which are autonomy-enhancing. Interventions must be ordered for efficient provision of care and the use of resources. The "line" itself has its own agendas and speed. The informed consent gained while the patient is being rolled down to the operating suite may well imply a lack of organization and sensitivity on the part of the clinician. But it also stems from the exigencies of the system. Within such a pace, this may well be the easiest point at which two birds can be killed with one stone—get the patient to the operating room and get his consent to what will happen there where a refusal would be contrary to the whole momentum of the situation and be increasingly unlikely. We cannot afford to have the operating room empty or have surgeons standing around with their hands in their pockets. There are surely better ways to do all this, but even still, the rhythm and pressure of such agendas will remain. And such focus will remain contrary to the autonomy of the patient who lacks understanding, is hesitant or worried, or might well have second thoughts if given the opportunity.

Add to all this the fact that the patient is like a fish out of water within an unfamiliar, often alien and seemingly bizarre environment. Surrounded by blinking lights, digital readouts, space age technology, and the institutional colors of the rainbow, the possibility that one mere human being could be self-determining within the belly of such a beast starts to take on long odds. It may well be that the legal presumption of competence is thus best construed *not* as a realistic belief in its presence and efficacy, but rather as a shrill insistence on its authority, given the myriad forces that would tend to overwhelm or supplant it. But since we are trying to be realistic, let us get the facts straight.

We are not just speaking of hospital-based, tertiary care. Similar assembly-line, efficiency-driven characteristics abound in clinics and private doctors' offices. If such enterprises want to pay their bills and earn a respectable profit, they simply cannot routinely engage in extensive discussions with most of their patients. Correlatively, patients who feel sick enough to come in for care, and may well have already spent a good deal of time sitting on their hands in the waiting room, seem no more inclined to play "medical consumer" when ushered into the doctor's presence than the patient being wheeled down to the operating room on a gurney. Finally, patients hardly need to be suffering from hypercalcemia secondary to end-stage cancer to be diminished in their actual capacity to attend to whatever information is presented or maintain their status as autonomous decision makers. Those who doubt this should reflect back on how they felt and what they did the last time they had the flu. Again, a spontaneous, sustained pursuit of patient understanding and autonomy is not going to tend to arise from either party.

The Nature of Clinical Decision Making

As if diminished competence and the anonymous medical assembly line were not enough, we have yet to reflect on the complexities that are often ingredient in the sorts of decisions informed consent is supposed to facilitate. As noted, many medical decisions may well be quite straightforward, with no real alternatives and a clear balance of benefit over risk. This is not always the case, and, particularly in those situations where basic values *are* at stake for the patient, the decision matrix may well present a much more opaque, inscrutable face. *The final barrier to patient autonomy lies in the decision itself.*

Begin with the uncertainties, possibilities, and probabilities inherent in many clinical situations. Next, add a viable alternative treatment or two with multiple branches for the decision tree depending on further diagnostic results, complications, or the degree to which the patient does or does not respond to initial interventions. Then, add the idiosyncrasies of the effects on and responses of individual patients to illness and treatment. Finally, place all this within a continually evolving clinical picture that might challenge the most experienced clinician. At some point we should surely wonder if talk of the "essentials" of the decision is not just a ridiculous shorthand for situations whose concurrent complexity, ambiguity, fluidity, and uncertainty admit of no clear, simple, or static vision. The technical language of the profession, which supposedly can have no place in informed consent, may then instead seem absolutely necessary for the project of conceptualization, not to mention evaluating and making decisions about what has thus been so precariously fashioned. But where, we must ask, does that leave the patient, assaulted by illness, a stranger in a strange land, when he finally steps up to the podium to render judgment?

SUMMARY REMARKS

For all the skepticism the preceding may raise about patient autonomy and informed consent, it is certainly not clear that basic public policy changes will flow from such findings. For one thing, my experience teaching undergraduate students in bioethics classes, who come from many different backgrounds and vocations, is that the preceding data and caveats are almost always met with a firm and jaundiced eye. However much one tries to identify the presence and sources of diminished competence, most students continue to reject the implication that patient autonomy may thus be a will-o'-the-wisp. The legal presumption of competence, with its low threshold and allied right to refuse treatment, is simply not a notion that students are willing to abandon, whatever the facts or arguments. The commentator who thus attempts to argue us back to the days of "doctor knows best" is being completely unrealistic about what the public and its elected representatives will accept. That ship has sailed.

In the same breath, one should also recognize the credibility that accrues to the clinician who remains lukewarm about such presumptions and pretense. The law may well mandate informed consent and enshrine the right to refuse treatment. The clinician then gets to respond with the informed consent ritual and a grudging acceptance of treatment refusals where counseling fails. But acquiescence to legal and societal conceits is one thing. A diligent, committed pursuit of them, particularly when they conflict with the clinician's daily experience *and* available time, is another. We are thus left to wonder if and when a conscientious physician is ever obliged to pursue patient autonomy and understanding in any forceful way. And, hopefully, the proponent of such patient autonomy will recognize that a conscientious pursuit by the clinician is absolutely crucial, given the preceding, if informed consent is to have a chance of being effective. Effective for what? It is high time we get much clearer about what goods and values informed consent might pursue, particularly as the enterprise now appears so ill-starred. Is there really that much at stake here, and if so, what? For, given that the enterprise seems so ill-starred, we are surely now obliged to make sure that it is somehow still justified.

NOTES

1. That such a counseling and clarificatory response is appropriate in the case where a patient rejects recommended therapy is clear from many studies indicating that the rejection of the treatment might well be due to such questionable factors as clinically treatable depression or the patient's significant misconceptions of his situation and prospects. See Jackson and Youngner, 1979, for the classic study of this problem.

2. If one were to simply average the results of past studies, the average would come out to around 50 percent recall of information provided. This is a very crude figure, however, as some studies focus on patient recall months after informed consent, as did Robinson and Merav, who found a 20 percent rate of recall (Robinson and Merav, 1976). Aside from falsely equating remembering after the fact with understanding at the point of consent, the significant effect of the normal forgetting process is well documented. Bengler et al., for example, found a 72 percent rate of recall at two hours past informed consent, and a 61 percent rate three months later (Bengler et al., 1980). Morgan and Schwab, for their part, tested immediately after consent and only received a 37 percent rate of recall (Morgan and Schwab, 1986). See especially Roth and Meisel's "What We Do and Do Not Know About Informed Consent" for an extended discussion of the problems and flaws of the extant studies, as well as the reasons why no clear implications seem to emerge from them. (Roth and Meisel, 1981). Interpretation of studies beyond 1981 would also be usefully preceded by a review of this article.

3. For a fairly exhaustive list of most of the existing studies, see the bibliography of Meisel, 1981. For whatever reason, the bulk of studies that actually document specific levels of patient understanding to informed consents

occurred in the 1970s and early 1980s; beyond that point there are few such studies (none of which give any detail as to what was asked, how it was tested, etc.) with much more attention to either patient perceptions of informed consent or patient satisfaction, neither of which helps us regarding actual understanding.

4. Cassileth et al., 1980, p. 896; Lidz, 1984, p. 318; see also Fellner and Marshall, 1970.

5. One could, of course, argue that the lack of careful reading of consent forms testifies to such a tendency in illness.

4

The Potential Benefits of Informed Consent

Our inquiry repeatedly tugs us back and forth. The law, rhetorically at least, advanced its doctrine of informed consent in terms of the fundamental principle of self-determination. Unfortunately, the law's specific focus has come to be on torts; and it thus provides little clear, specific guidance regarding how informed consent should actually pursue such self-determination. Concurrently, the law tends to induce behaviors in clinicians that are counterproductive to such a pursuit— for example, the hyperinforming that leads to information overload. The new ethos of patient autonomy, for its part, enjoys broad societal consensus regarding many of its basic prescriptions. Further, like the law, the new ethos seems to presume that certain needs as well as patient abilities are usually present in the same form and degree. But such univocal presumptions regarding patient abilities and needs clearly run afoul of clinical experience and its supporting empirical literature. The icing on the cake is then supplied by reflecting on the diminishment of and barriers to autonomy that are ingredient in the situation of illness and health care, especially when we think of the "essay mode" of understanding, which is surely what we should hope for.

Whether, and in what form and degree, informed consent should be mandated for all clinical encounters thus remains quite unclear. It will probably continue to be legally required in countries like America, given societal attitudes and what now amounts to a strong legal tradition. But such a requirement does not address the issue of what, beyond some self-protective ritual, a conscientious clinician should be pursuing when he offers a given patient informed consent. Clinicians have the right and need to inquire as to what such an intervention might really be worth, why they should bother with it. And if the reply is no more than that the law requires it, or that it is supported by strong societal expectations, then given the preceding critique of the

66

assumptions surrounding informed consent and patient autonomy, one can hardly fault the clinician who gives informed consent only a ritualistic observance and moves on to other matters.

It is thus time to pick up the gauntlet cast down by the paternalist in chapter 2. The paternalist's challenge remains the pertinent one— namely, what, on the score of a given patient's actual and significant needs, might realistically be pursued by the provision of informed consent? What goods and values might it actually capture and how do these vary, in importance and availability, from patient to patient? In sum, is informed consent an intervention that might effectively and efficiently change outcomes for the better and if so, which outcomes, when, and for whom?

This work will thus proceed as though all the theoretical arguments and insights regarding autonomy and freedom are insufficient for a comprehensive appreciation of informed consent. Instead, our argument will key to the traditional principle of *beneficence*—that is, the patient's best interests. With this focus, we thus place the debate about informed consent within the context of the realities, needs, and actual opportunities of the physician-patient encounter. Remembering that we are speaking of a doctrine that its proponents want to institute for all clinical encounters, and that its core agenda relates to patient participation in decision making, we must first inquire whether this goal is, in fact, always present in any meaningful sense.

THE VALUE OF PATIENT PARTICIPATION IN MEDICAL DECISION MAKING

Informed consent may make various contributions, but its core and most controversial function lies in the notion of patients actually participating in medical decision making. And it is here that the autonomist and the clinician most tend to butt heads. The autonomist insists that any intervention merits informed consent, as there is *always* the choice between performing it or not. The clinician may quickly retort that many medical interventions are so clearly indicated that no such decision making on the patient's part is needed.

Now it is appropriate to recognize that chronic and terminal illness calls for counseling toward enhancing insight and adaptive responses. Major risks, limitations, or uncertainties of interventions merit disclosure, and compliance must be stimulated. Equally, matters of profound and personal significance to the patient may need to be weighed and decided in specific cases. But none of the above are *always* at issue. It is often the case that no major life choices are at stake, the risks are relatively insignificant, and the benefits of a given intervention are clear and compelling. And thus those who insist on the importance of patient participation in decision making in *all* cases are, with respect to the common clinical situation, grossly exaggerating the needs and tasks at hand.

The autonomist response here might be that if there is any risk to the intervention at all, or if the benefit might not occur, then the patient deserves to be informed regardless of how "clearly indicated" the intervention is. Equally, if the benefit itself has limitations, complications, or side effects that are likely to disappoint or discomfort the patient, such realities also merit mention. If the clinician is offering an intervention with no risks, complications, or side effects, the benefits of which are instantaneous, certain to occur, and without any limitations, and which is substantially preferable to doing nothing at all, then one might well wonder what the content of the choice is. But aside from there being few such ideal interventions, the autonomist may respond by wondering why the clinician might not enjoy so describing such a paragon of treatment to his patient. And to the extent the treatment at issue departs from such ideal conditions, the clinician will have a bit more to say.

Fair enough. But a problem arises for the clinician in situations where he would justifiably see a given treatment as "clearly indicated." In such cases it is rather strange to suggest that the physician should approach the patient as if he really had a decision to participate in, or that a subsequent refusal should be seen as an exercise in personal autonomy, not a cause for alarm (or suggestive of patient incompetence).

The way out here is to hold that patient autonomy and informed consent in such situations are, at least in the core sense of the patient's participating in medical decisions, theoretical concerns that merit only minimal effort. In effect a relatively brief, noninteractive ritual presentation might be quite sufficient in certain cases. Thus, as a treatment approaches the ideal "clearly indicated" case, such participation gets increasingly trivial, and both patient and physician might well legitimately feel they have much more important tasks before them.

Clinically, there is another way to put the preceding. Say the clinician approaches his patient with a recommendation that he feels is clearly indicated. We may tentatively define such a situation as follows: the patient definitely does not want to simply grin and bear his illness, the treatment is successful in most cases, it has a clear and substantial advantage over any alternative modalities, its benefits are clearly and substantially superior to the complex of possible complications and side effects that attend it, and there is no significant threat of chronic or terminal illness with attendant informational, counseling, or adaptive needs.

Now an informed consent ritual in such cases could satisfy the law. This ritual could also function as a rule-out procedure whereby the hesitant, fearful, risk-aversive patient can identify himself and trigger further discussion. But what if the physician strongly suspects that the patient is not even listening to the ritual, as clinical experience and the empirical literature suggests may often be the case? Is it appropriate for the physician to pause and say to the patient, "Look, we have an important decision to make, and you don't seem to be even listening to me. Let's go over it one more time, attentively!"? Further, is it also appropriate for the physician, beyond any present dictate of the law, to attempt to test the patient's actual understanding of his situation and prospects? And if this is marginal, or worse, or the patient just says "C'mon, doc, just do what you think is best," should the physician pause for a soliloquy on the virtues of patient autonomy?

I submit that none of the above behaviors are indicated as there may be no significant decision-making goal that merits pursuit in such "clearly indicated treatment" situations. The patient's *authorization* of treatment needs to be solicited. Equally, the ritual presentation of informed consent for informational and rule-out purposes provides an opportunity to identify problems or hesitations on the patient's part. If the patient does not indicate any such problems, and the physician sees none either, then the autonomist will perhaps allow our participants to proceed, without further harassment, to the treatment that the patient came for and that the physician is eager to provide. Such an allowance by the autonomist may well be forthcoming, but it must be noted as a substantial one. Such an allowance accepts the idea that patient participation in medical decision making is not *always* a significant clinical goal. Depending on one's perspective, it can arguably result in the perception that such participation is not even commonly a significant clinical agenda as clinicians tend to see many interventions as clearly indicated.

We will have to reflect further on when an intervention is clearly indicated. Surely this is a designation that an informed, competent patient might disagree with his physician about. At this juncture, however, our point need only be that patient participation in decision making may well not be a major agenda in a significant number of cases. Thus we have not yet identified a *major* value that is *always* at stake in clinical encounters.

Given the preceding, we might more fruitfully turn the tables here and ask: when is it the case that such patient participation *is* important in treatment decisions? A number of answers seem legitimate. (1) It is always important when the patient, by means of treatment refusal, hesitancy, further questions, or the expression of doubts or fears, indicates that it is. (2) It is also important to the degree the patient's situation and prospects depart from the "clearly indicated" picture previously mentioned. Is there an alternative treatment that is arguably less risky or attended by less pain and suffering, though it may not be as effective as the one the physician is recommending? Choices between medical and surgical management often seem to incorporate such trade-offs. Is one treatment more attractive as far as mortality rates go, but less on the score of morbidity, particularly in the long term? A patient might validly opt for an alternative procedure that, though it does not offer the best life expectancy, does offer a life that is less battered or diminished by treatment. The debates over medical versus surgical management of chronic heart disease provide pertinent examples of choices that adequately informed patients might well evaluate quite differently. Somewhere between single- and triple-vessel disease, the choice between angioplasty and coronary artery bypass graft seems to turn mainly on whether the patient is talking to an internist or a surgeon. But such major high-stakes interventions should be evaluated in terms of more than whether the patient's physician tends to prefer pills to the knife, or vice versa. And once one has heard these parties discuss their preferences face to face, it becomes apparent that there are serious issues concerning types and degrees of morbidity, as well as the possibility and extent of long-term cure, that are at stake. But these sorts of factors are precisely those that patients tend to evaluate differently if given the opportunity. Cancer patients, equally, often face such choices, and the physician who does not apprise them of such choices robs them of their freedom as surely as if he had lied to them.

Again, however, we must wonder how actively the physician should pursue patient participation in such instances. What if the patient remains unwilling to step up to the podium of judgment?

Many often balk at this, either out of conflicting needs for reassurance and maintaining hope or from beliefs in physicians' expertise and their own lack of it. Should the physician attempt to drag them to the water even when they do not appear thirsty? The physician should identify significant choices, but should he encourage reflection and choice at such junctures? This depends on numerous factors, including the significance and poignancy of the choice, the patient's degree of interest in or aversion to participating in it, and the degree to which the choice at hand can be meaningfully and adequately rendered for the particular patient. In sum, there appear to be numerous variables even when important choices exist.

There are also situations in which the physician cannot legitimately make a recommendation to the patient without substantial input from him. There are situations when the values at stake are so profound and personal that only the patient can speak to them. The physician who makes a recommendation in such cases is simply ignoring the possibility that the patient's values may differ radically from his own. One clear example would be an elective termination of pregnancy. Another would be the situation in which conventional treatment for a cancer patient has failed and the alternative to no further treatment involves an experimental protocol with major morbidity that offers a small chance of cure or long-term remission but would, if unsuccessful, simply result in the destruction of the remaining good time the patient has left if he chose palliation instead. A final example would be the patient in end-stage renal failure who is faced with a choice between the mortality of a renal transplant and the morbidity of dialysis.

There is thus a spectrum of cases ranging from those in which the patient may acceptably remain silent and let the physician speak to those where the physician should remain silent until the patient speaks. Sometimes patient autonomy is absolutely necessary, sometimes only a generic permission or authorization is enough, and often the situation falls in between, depending on numerous variables. A universal ritual calibrates to none of this, but neither does skepticism about informed consent when such profoundly individual choices appear. Theoretically there is always a choice, often this choice is a significant one, and the physician should at least identify the choice to the patient, if not insist that he grapple with it. Often the patient's response, at least as a decision-making act, will amount to no more than acceptance of the physician's recommendations. The common one-way communication at the bedside may thus be quite satisfactory in many cases. In other cases, a true dialogue is needed. That the law captures none of this variability, and the new ethos proceeds as if it did not exist by insisting on patient autonomy at the institution of any new therapy, is part of what we are grappling with here.

GOODS AND VALUES THAT INFORMED CONSENT MIGHT CAPTURE

We should next inquire whether there are goods and values other than patient participation in decision making that are always at issue in clinical encounters. Given that such decision making is the core meaning of informed consent, this is a departure from the usual agenda. We will thus be speaking of goals that might be pursued by tactics other than informed consent, however much it might be one way of gaining them or be foundational to such an effort. *Are there any significant goals, other than those directly keyed to patient decision making, that informed consent might pursue in every physician-patient encounter?*

It turns out that there are quite a few of them. (1) It could assist in developing the physician-patient relationship beyond the aforementioned "moral strangers" state. Even if such an enhanced relationship is unlikely to be significant in the current situation, it might well be at another time—for example, when the need to address advanced directives presents itself. (2) To the extent the benefits of and prognosis with treatment may fall short of the ideal of full and timely restoration of function, the patient can be led to a more realistic appreciation of his situation and prospects. Such an appreciation would also tend to protect the viability of the physician-patient relationship if the results were, in fact, less than what had been hoped for. (3) Even the abstract presentation of the choice between treatment and no intervention at all might serve to instruct the patient that such an activity on his part can be an important activity within the clinical encounter. Perhaps some diminishment of the urge to be passive and assume that doctor always knows best could occur. Such a result could be of value at another time when patient understanding and participation *are* important. (4) Particularly if interactive, the patient being queried as to what characteristics and effects his problem has, the communication process could also (a) assist the physician in seeing what personal meanings the patient's problem has in his life, (b) assist in identifying the subtly but functionally incompetent patient, (c) identify and respond to any significant misconceptions, false hopes, or fears that the patient may have, and (d) stimulate the patient to be more forthcoming with information, thus enhancing the quality of the history and workup in terms more specific to that particular patient.

Nor is this all. Surely one way to provide patients the reassurance they seek is to have the physician diagnose and explain their condition and his plans for treating it. Simply labeling the disease turns some nameless threat into something that is known and may now be dealt with. The clinician thereby can establish himself as an advocate and guide within the otherwise threatening medical assembly line. Equally, concern and compassion can be expressed in the specific terms of the patient's actual problems, not just by some abstract hand holding or similar gestures that have no anchor in the patient's life. What better way to announce that help has arrived? Potentially counterproductive anxiety can thus be diminished, acceptance of and commitment to a treatment regimen gained, compliance, cooperation, and self-monitoring stimulated. Even if the clinician sees no sense in which a real choice is at hand, all these are treatment-enhancing goals, and one might wonder if there is a better way to pursue them than in terms of a cogent explanation of the problem at hand and the planned response to it.

Such a communication process can thus enhance *any therapeutic encounter* and have value in developing the physician-patient relationship. It will also aid in the pursuit of diagnostic and therapeutic goals. As far as patient participation in decision making goes, this activity may have little real place in many interventions, but a basic rendition of the risks and benefits could serve a rule-out sort of function by tending to identify the patient who has idiosyncratic fears, misconceptions, or hesitations regarding medical care in general. Surely such factors merit identification up front and might well be easily identified and rectified. Finally, it is a commonplace that mention of the significant risks of any intervention will tend to diminish the risk of suit for the clinician, not only by fulfilling the legal requirement but, hopefully, by also instilling in the patient a corresponding sense that he has chosen the intervention and thus feels some personal responsibility for this choice.

Substantial Goods and Values That Are Often at Stake

If we thus depart from the usual "patient participation in decision making" emphasis of the new ethos, it turns out that there are numerous significant clinical goals that informed consent might pursue. The trick is to recognize that informed consent can also be effective to other goals that any experienced clinician would tend to value. It does not just address a decision-making activity that often has little or no clinical credibility. Having serious clinical doubts about patient engagement in the "essay mode" of decision making thus in no way damns the informed consent enterprise. Numerous other goals, which do not require such a level of understanding and reflection, are often at stake. Such goals are more informational. The patient needs to get some sense of the source of his problem and what can be done about it. If the results are likely to be other than immediate, of limited effect with a chronic residue, gained at the cost of a significant convalescent period, or come with certain adverse side effects, temporary or permanent, then the viability of the physician-patient relationship requires that the patient actually recognize them as soon as possible. The empirical literature suggests that this may require significant, repeated effort. Other positive effects have already been noted: (1) the anticipation of expected pain and discomfort tends to diminish its effect; (2) to the extent the problem stems from self-destructive patient behaviors, preventive goals can be pursued; (3) the patient can be apprised of possible chronic effects on his lifestyle and assisted to plan for these; and (4) the clinician can often enhance the possibility of successful treatment by generating a knowledgeable, committed, even optimistic patient, which in turn can yield dividends in patient compliance, cooperation, and self-monitoring.

Equally, an interactive process can identify fear, confusion, anxiety, and misconceptions on the patient's part. These factors will not be uncovered by a ritualistic, one-sided offering of informed consent. But they surely merit identification and response since they may well cause the patient more suffering than any treatment or disease will produce.[1] Further, patients' initial perceptions of their problem and its potential resolutions are *likely* to be wide of the mark. They may be overly apprehensive in a situation where treatment will probably be successful. Conversely, they may fail to appreciate the significance of the threat to them, or of the effort required to remove it. The clinician might often dispel such sources of counterproductive and harmful behavior in patients, particularly before they have time to fester. A little extra time spent soliciting the patient's sense of the nature and effects of his problem will provide the groundwork for such an intervention.

Less Common but Profound Goods and Values

Eric Cassell's point that often the best way to protect or restore the patient's autonomy is to cure the patient should always be borne in mind in discussions such as these (Cassell, 1977). Thus, what the patient came for, and what the physician is trained to provide—that is, treatment—remains where it belongs, at center stage. The point of the preceding is thus not to usurp center stage. Rather, it is to make sure that the play is not conducted by one actor in a monotone.

But special needs, at times far more important than any treatment regimen, arise in certain types of cases, especially where chronic or terminal illness threatens the patient. A number of these variable needs have already been noted: (1) the need for the patient to understand, ponder, and pass on major, eminently personal, implications of their treatment and further care; (2) the patient's need to grasp and adapt to profound effects on his lifestyle and expectations given the presence of chronic or terminal illness; and (3) assisting the patient, who because of pain, abandonment, or situational depression has tended to give up hope and control. Institutionalized patients come particularly to mind with their oft-noted childlike deterioration. Such deterioration can be particularly counterproductive in situations where the difference between success or failure may turn on the patient's coping and adaptive responses to a reduced quality or expected duration of life. *In sum, the protection or restoration of patient autonomy may, at times, need to occupy center stage and be preparatory and foundational to all other goals.* It does little good to enhance function or extend life if the patient is indisposed to value or take advantage of it. And at times the primary goal will relate to objectives that only the patient can address: active participation in rehabilitation, major modifications and acceptance of a lifestyle imbedded in chronic illness, or the performance of "last things" to the extent terminal illness threatens. Few of us do such things well; many stumble and falter. Informed consent, far beyond the legal ritual, allied with referrals to self-help groups, community assistance, and counseling services, can make all the difference.

Other needs arise in such situations. (1) Knowledgeable patients will be better able to reflect about the degree of aggressiveness of treatment they desire, and how and where they wish to spend their remaining time. They will also tend to more effectively address the issues involved in formulating a living will or designating a proxy toward the possibility that such treatment might be either limited or discontinued at a certain point. The patient who has been kept informed from the beginning, however modest or circumscribed the initial information, is better prepared to deal with such profound matters. One must question the so-called "compassion" that keeps physicians from sharing their deeper fears with patients early on. Such "compassion" is false in two senses: (a) it appears to be done more toward the goal of avoiding a disagreeable discussion, and (b) it often results in much more suffering down the line, either because the patient was not given the chance to rule out aggressive treatment that he would not have wanted, or because he is unprepared to do so from lack of anticipation. (2) Some patients with self-destructive lifestyles (e.g., nicotine or alcohol abuse) seem much more approachable at the point of their first major hospitalization. The clinician can sometimes generate an about-face in behavior that television messages or advice in the office setting often cannot. (3) The role of families can also be addressed, enlisting them in patient counseling and the provision of alternative care in the home situation, and assisting them to see the often significant effects on their own lives that chronic or terminal illness in a loved one may bring.

RETROSPECT AND PROSPECT

Much more could be written about any of the previous needs and agendas, whether we are speaking of formulating patient preferences regarding aggressiveness of treatment (King, 1991), concerned with assisting a patient to fashion adaptive responses to chronic illness, or attempting to deal with noncompliant or self-destructive behavior. For our purposes at this juncture, however, the following points merit emphasis: (1) that no legal ritual or formula can address such a spectrum of variable agendas; (2) skepticism regarding patient autonomy on the basis of clinical experience may have its place, but it cannot be allowed to dictate clinician behavior—too much of importance will fail to be addressed if this is allowed; and (3) informed consent and allied behaviors by the clinician are important clinical activities, depending on numerous variables in the patient's situation and capacities.

Conceptually, we are thus left with the conclusion that there exists a heterogeneity of needs and opportunities that informed consent might pursue, depending on the patient and the situation at hand. At one extreme, these needs can be quickly met, accomplished by what amounts to a one-way, noninteractive ritual of information provision. Concurrently, there may be no significant sense in which the patient has any choice to make, however important it is for him to signal acceptance of the clinician's plan of action. At the other extreme, substantial needs may be present that demand that informed consent and allied tactics occupy center stage. There may well be decisions that only the patient can speak to, as well as adaptive and anticipatory responses that can only be accomplished by the person at risk. In between these extremes, diverse needs and possibilities merit various types and degrees of response. Which is to say what we might well have expected from the beginning—namely, that each patient is unique in this area, as in any other, and competent, effective medical care must be responsive to such uniqueness.

Clinician skepticism regarding such enterprises can be healthy or malignant. A healthy skepticism surely will combat the Pelagian sort of heresy that patients can attain insight in illness without assistance.[2] Neither the law nor the new ethos seems to have a sufficient sense of this, and it is their deepest failing. In such matters, *the unassisted patient is an abandoned patient.* Clinician skepticism can also assist the clinician in recognizing when such goals are trivial or unattainable. The ethical provision of scarce and expensive medical care—that is, the clinician's time—also must focus on the clinician's pursuit of those outcomes that are most valuable and attainable. In this sense, patient autonomy becomes one value among numerous others and should be allowed to trump nothing.

Conversely, clinician skepticism becomes malignant when it inappropriately discounts the preceding sorts of goals and clings to a technical, medical model of care as if patients were not people at all but bodies lacking any spiritual dimension or uniqueness in their own right. Contemporary medicine has tended to do just this, and such a critique is the most basic feedback that it is receiving from its charges. And, to the extent the profession remains rogue and insensitive in this regard, it has no basis for complaint when the law steps in. *None* of the goals stressed in this chapter should come as a surprise to any experienced clinician. They are obvious components of the fabric of illness and care. The task of the profession is to identify and respond to such goals and rising societal concerns, spontaneously and with the clinical nuance that only it can supply.

Toward assisting with this task, this work will now move on to provide an operational model of informed consent that has the

requisite flexibility, realism, and effectiveness that the preceding
analysis calls for. The solution to our dialectic here is not another
new theoretical perspective. Rather, it is the formulation of a management tool that will capture the preceding tensions and agendas,
effectively and efficiently addressing true patient needs while not
wasting time on the trivial, unattainable, or ancillary.

NOTES

1. See Cassell (1982) regarding a more clinically nuanced sense of suffering that includes the effects of uncertainty and corrosive worry.

2. The Pelagian heresy held that people could attain salvation by their
own efforts, without the assistance of grace. Our argument here concerning
patients' exercising freedom and autonomy in illness, as well as gaining
insight into their situation and prospects, challenges a similar error: the assistance of physicians in such tasks approaches that of a necessary condition.

PART II

A Model of
Informed Consent

5

Toward a Model of Informed Consent—Theoretical and Programmatic Considerations

What began as the "doctrine" of informed consent has now become the "problem" of informed consent. The possibility of successfully pursuing the goals and values of informed consent seems to recede just as these goods and values become clearer. Chapter 3 surely affords us no grounds for optimism. Even on a "bits and pieces" model of informed consent, many patients perform only marginally. If we move to the "essay mode" of understanding, we may well wonder how often this ideal is even remotely approached by most patients. And if we then include our reflections on diminished competence, the barriers to informed consent, and the complexities that medical decisions often present, the whole enterprise comes to look quite ill-starred.

The option of medical paternalism fares no better, however. As repeatedly noted, it offends against basic aspirations and assumptions of free men and women. The ship wherein physicians exercise unlimited authority over their charges has long since sailed. Further, goods and values that are crucial to the successful treatment of patients are at issue. Trust, acceptance, and understanding are foundational to compliance and cooperation, and the chronically and terminally ill need assistance appreciating profound events in their lives if "treatment" is to be more than a quite temporary and quickly ineffective bandaid.

We may well wonder at this juncture if our "problem" is intractable; that this may be the case can be brought into fuller relief by reflecting further on the ways in which our problem presents both intellectual and practical conundrums.

We should easily be able to imagine any number of extended further debates issuing from the discussions through which one attempts to gain a coherent formulation to solve the problem. The sort of dialectic that took place in chapter 2 could easily start anew. The proponents of patient autonomy might well fault the preceding as too disparaging of patients, as well as provide further detail and emphasis to the findings of the previous chapter. They might also attempt to recast the notion of autonomy at the bedside by fashioning a much richer and more flexible concept of it, instructed by the goods and values identified in the previous chapter, as well as by the sobering message of its predecessor. Those who remain skeptical about informed consent, for their part, might want to further emphasize the pessimistic implications of chapter 3. In this regard, the ethical principle of "should implies can" might be utilized toward the point that however valuable the goods and values arrayed in chapter 4, substantial grounds for doubt exist as to whether they can be efficiently and effectively pursued.

The "problem" of informed consent is also practical. We began with a relatively simple and static conception of informed consent in the law, where patient competence is to be presumed and the types of information to be disclosed are clear. But we have come to see that there are so many variables in any given case that a generic model of informed consent will be either insufficiently detailed or overwhelmingly byzantine. The previous chapter describes a complex spectrum or heterogeneity of goods and values in this area. In some cases, there may well be little or no sense in which there are important choices at hand (e.g., when ampicillin-sensitive pneumonia is diagnosed). In other situations, such as newly discovered metastatic disease, choices of profound and personal moment are unavoidable, and detailed insight into one's situation and prospects are essential. Similarly, patient competence to understand and participate in medical decision making comes in a spectrum, from the essentially nonexistent to the marginal to the well-informed and reflective. A patient's place within this spectrum will be more or less acceptable depending on the case and actual needs at hand. Finally, any of the other goods and values just identified will be variously significant and attainable from case to case, patient to patient. The experienced clinician might well conclude that the complexities of a differential diagnosis will often look simple compared with what is being contemplated here.

This book will not fully resolve the "problem" of informed consent in either of the two preceding senses. On an intellectual level, we will not renew the dialectic that occurred in chapter 2. Such a discussion could well remain inconclusive, or at least rob us of space better spent providing detail to an operational model. Further, whatever new, more multifactorial definition of autonomy we might be able to formulate, instructed and limited by the preceding reflections, the basic question would still remain: how and in what specific senses might such goods and values be captured at the bedside? Intellectual progress at a theoretical level would thus do little to dispel clinician skepticism at the bedside.

Equally, the practical problem of providing a comprehensive and nuanced model of informed consent cannot be fully pursued in this work. Every type of intervention, as well as patient circumstance, will come with its own unique possibilities and complexities, and be further complicated by the special capacities, interests, and needs of the patient at hand. No model is going to remove the need for judgment calls at the bedside, or the possibility that well-intentioned people can legitimately see matters differently. Nor can it provide a cookbook approach as to how any individual situation should be addressed.

Given its clinician readership, this work will recast the "problem" of informed consent at this point into a more clinically appropriate form: granted that we have identified goods and values of significant clinical and ethical moment, which may or may not be present in a given clinical encounter, is there some generic model that can be seen as credibly pursuing such values? And "credibly" is the operative word. To be a credible model, particularly for practicing clinicians, it must be seen as providing for an efficient and effective pursuit of such goals, without wasting time or becoming distracted by the pursuit of the ancillary or unattainable.

The problem of informed consent will thus be approached in this work as if it is a Gordian knot that will not admit of an intellectual unraveling but must be severed by a practical resolution that incorporates and responds to relevant goals, possibilities, and variables *for the most part*. The nature of this severing may be received as follows. Informed consent is not just a doctrine; it is equally and for our purposes, primarily, an *intervention intended to change outcomes*. Which outcomes? The first answer is that this depends on the case at hand. But our model cannot be this flexible; there are certain goods and values that we generally expect will be at issue in most clinical encounters, and others that are important enough, although less often present, that we at least need to monitor or somehow provide for them. Minimally, we need to provide the patient sufficient detail regarding his situation, prospects, and the choice at hand so that he can meaningfully *authorize* his physician to proceed. We have also identified the need for the patient to rule himself in or out regarding hesitation, ambivalence, or misconceptions regarding the proposed course of therapy. Such a rule-out itself requires significant detail, as well as some sort of efficient feedback mechanism. Further, we have identified certain issues that are not always present in a consent situation but that must be monitored for, the most important of these being whether the patient is competent to consent to treatment. Some monitoring of the patient's competence, at least in the sense that we will be triggered to investigate it further in appropriate cases, must be included. Finally, although we have downplayed the idea that patients will commonly desire or need to seek full understanding of their situation and prospects, we should still provide some groundwork for such understanding in case the patient either desires this or needs to attain it in special circumstances—for example, when "profound and personal" choices are at hand.

Some goods and values will thus always be provided for in our model, some will be anticipated to some degree in case they are present, some will be monitored so further response can be provided when indicated, and some will be pursued only if one of the two parties in the clinical encounter sees the need. And the "proof" of our resolution, agreement as to whether we have actually severed the Gordian knot of informed consent, will arise from the credibility of this model's approach to and provision for the goods and values already identified, credibility in large part being an integral function of efficiency and effectiveness. In sum, does the model pursue significant goods and values in any given case, and does it do this in a way that avoids wasting time pursuing the ancillary and unattainable, thereby providing an efficient intervention?

This model will be provided in the next three chapters, first by articulating the sorts of content and structure an informed consent should typically have, then by a discussion of the nature of patient competence relating especially to how it will be assessed, and finally by a review of the basic exceptions to informed consent that have been advocated, such as the emergency exception.

We must first, however, clarify what it means to provide such a model; we cannot escape the intellectual problem altogether. In part this will be accomplished by placing this work within the context of certain prior theoretical discussions of informed consent. We must also further specify what amounts to the basic theoretical neutrality of this book—that certain claims or arguments will *not* be used to generate or support our results. As already stated, the "proof" of our model will be a practical one: does it credibly provide for and pursue the goods and values identified? We will finally need to canvass certain basic choices regarding the form and focus of this model—for example, whether informed consent will typically occur as a discrete event or be offered more as a process occurring over time.

THEORETICAL CONSIDERATIONS AND COMMITMENTS

A number of works offer general accounts or theories regarding the nature of informed consent. This work must be situated within that literature. This discussion occurs here, rather than earlier on, because the differences between this work and others can be coherently seen only in terms of the previous chapters and the problem that has emerged from them.

The Theory of Informed Consent of Faden and Beauchamp

One work merits separate reference in this regard, both because it is the best-known contemporary discussion of informed consent and because, though it is a particularly theoretical work, it specifically anticipates the more practical enterprise in which we are engaged. Ruth Faden and Tom Beauchamp, in their work *A History and Theory of Informed Consent*, have provided the most searching, sustained, and philosophically sophisticated discussion of informed consent to date (Faden and Beauchamp, 1986). The first part of their work offers a detailed historical account of the notion of informed consent, both within the tradition of the medical profession (e.g., as expressed in ancient writings and modern codes) and as a developing principle in the law. They then proceed, in the latter part of the work, to offer a theory of informed consent. It is important for us to clarify what their theory does and does not provide.

As a theory, Faden and Beauchamp's offering, primed by legal and historical materials, is a tour de force of conceptual analysis. By conceptual analysis, I particularly mean the articulation of the meanings and implications of various key principles and characteristics ingredient in the doctrine of informed consent. What, for example, do such notions as competence, autonomy, understanding, and intention amount to, particularly with reference to the informed consent enterprise? What, given an analysis of these notions and the informed consent context, are useful guidelines for identifying and evaluating the possible goals and tactics of this enterprise and what might be identified as departures from it? Insights and assistance from such quarters as action theory, decision analysis, and contemporary psychology abound.

It must be emphasized, however, that for all the above, the authors explicitly deny that they are providing an operational model of informed consent; their work should not be seen as an attempt to solve the problem facing us. Little reference is made, for example, to the sobering message of the empirical literature. The authors have explicitly provided a historical and conceptual account of informed consent, not a normative one (Faden and Beauchamp, 1986, p. vii). They do not presume to have provided "an analysis of the desirability of participation by patients or subjects in decision-making, nor do we identify the conditions under which health care professionals and research investigators should obtain informed consents. We discuss the nature of informed consent, its conditions, and the ends it serves, but not whether and when informed consent obligations should be imposed" (Faden and Beauchamp, 1986, pp. vii–viii).

What are we to make of such a disclaimer? Is their discussion merely a "thought experiment"? When the authors refer to their offering as "a theory," do they mean to suggest that it is just one possible view among many others and can be evaluated only regarding its internal coherence? What of its relevance and usefulness in grappling with the problem that emerges from the preceding chapters or, more basically, in assisting the clinician who is attempting to determine what an ethically valid informed consent might be?

The authors are not so humble or frivolous. They clearly believe that they have correctly articulated the core meanings of the concept of informed consent, as well as its history, and assert that these are "directly relevant" to the "development of satisfactory policies and practices of informed consent." As they say, "there is a need to be clear concerning that about which we speak before reaching conclusions about how things ought to be" (Faden and Beauchamp, 1986, p. viii).

We should not fault the authors for thus intentionally limiting the scope of their discussion. We will have occasion to draw upon their insights and offerings repeatedly through the rest of this work. Equally, though we might well want to insist that the meaning of a concept is not some Platonic form, available for consideration without reference to its character and embodiment in the real world, the authors have done us a crucial service by displaying the meanings, interrelations, and implications of core notions at issue. We have spent the first part of this work attempting to articulate the various goals and alternative perspectives that may be taken on informed consent, particularly as a matter of law, ethics, and public policy. To attempt to offer an operational model of informed consent without reference or response to such materials would be simply frivolous. Here Faden and Beauchamp's work can be seen as complementary since they have articulated a standard by which an operational model can be judged: does it provide a coherent and philosophically sophisticated account that does justice to the meanings of the notions that we will be obliged to pass on? Not that there is any particular sanctity to such meanings. We may well be forced to make our own modifications or substitutions as we now move from "conceptual analysis" and the sources of the notion of informed consent to the task of determining what it should actually be at the bedside. Coherence of formulation we are bound to, being creative with terminology requires candor, caution, and precision, but present meanings of informed consent, as well as the more "political" sources of it, are hardly sacrosanct.

This work differs from that of Faden and Beauchamp in that it speaks precisely to the domain that they did not address—namely, what informed consent *should* actually come to at the bedside. They, in fact, anticipate just such a project and the different character it would have. They recognize that, *as a matter of public policy*, what we might actually require will turn on (1) considerations of "efficiency and effectiveness," (2) "what is fair and reasonable to require of health care professionals," *not* just on (3) what conceptual analysis has determined to be the "demands of a set of abstract conditions" (Faden and Beauchamp, 1986, p. 285). Elsewhere, they also anticipate a point that we will eventually need to make much of: having proposed various strategies for enhancing patient understanding, they conclude by emphasizing that they make "no normative claim" that such strategies *ought* to be used or should be legally mandated. Aside from the self-imposed limitations of the book, they note that this is so because "some of these strategies" may well take "a substantial amount of that scarcest of resources—the professional's time and the subject's or patient's time," and they prudently recognize that such expenditures "may not be warranted" in the case of "many less consequential procedures and interventions" (Faden and Beauchamp, 1986, p. 329).

Different cases present choices of varying degrees of consequence or importance and may correspondingly merit different levels of effort and assessment, given considerations of efficiency, effectiveness, and the prudent use of resources. And herein lies the different orientation of our attempt to fashion an operational model of informed consent, as opposed to conceptual analysis, even though the former is guided by the latter, of which it is the completion.

Theoretical Commitments and Biases of This Work

The reader may note the absence in this text of any chapter that provides an "introduction to ethics." It proceeds by assuming that its reader is sufficiently aware of basic ethical terminology and perspectives, and simply directs the reader to a few of the innumerable standard presentations of such materials in case the reader feels a need for such instruction.[1]

Certain specific theoretical commitments and biases guide this work, however, and these should be explicated up front as we move from exposition and dialectic to sustained argument for and elaboration of a specific operational model. Such an explication will first be accomplished negatively here by noting certain theoretical sorts of arguments that this work will *not* utilize. In sum, by embracing a practical approach to severing the Gordian knot facing us, we also embrace an essentially theory-neutral view.

Ethical Theory

This work arises out of no specific primary allegiance to any particular ethical theory, nor does its argument appeal for support from such a ground. It recognizes no a priori first principles, and will thus not offer any purely deductive arguments from such sources. In appreciating this work, rule utilitarianism might best be taken to describe its approach and type of finding, particularly in its concern for consequences, efficiency, and effectiveness, and the formulation of rules of thumb to guide and habituate certain behaviors. But it will be equally concerned to identify appropriate departures from and exceptions to such guidelines.

We should also acknowledge principles that may be regarded as deontological, however, at least in the sense that they arise from more than a simply utilitarian consideration of consequences. The right not to be deceived and the right not to be treated against one's will are both supportable by a Kantian reflection on the nature of the rights and requisite respect for persons.[2] It should also be emphasized, however, that such deontological principles are negative sorts of rights, requiring only forbearance by others; they are not positive rights that place specific duties on others. The pertinent example of the latter sort of positive right—the right to an informed consent—will *not* be treated as deontologically based. As we noted in chapter 2, there may well be rights to refuse treatment, as well as not to be deceived or treated without one's permission. Whether or not a health care provider is also obliged to seek such permission with some presentation of the nature of the choice at hand is thus seen as a matter of values and consequences, of possible societal requirements and commitments that, ethically, need not necessarily be embraced for any straightforward a priori reason. In sum, this work will not attempt to resolve the "problem" of informed consent simply by insisting on some ideal principle. Its argument is beneficence-based, resting on the goods and values identified in chapter 4. And it will further proceed by accepting the challenge that an efficient and effective clinical model must be supplied for the pursuit of such goods and values. We will, in sum, meet the paternalist on his own ground, rather than attempt some theoretical end run around him.

Rights

This author also believes that there has been a marked deterioration in the realm of ethical discourse, particularly in the usage of "rights" language. The special status we have traditionally given to rights has been contaminated by the addition of many other "rights" that should better be seen as basic "claims" that people tend to make. Again, the pertinent example is the "right to informed consent," which should hardly be approached as having the same status as *negative forbearance rights,* such as the rights to life, liberty, and the pursuit of happiness. The latter are, I believe, mandatory for any decent society and are particularly noncontroversial as they place no positive duties upon others, only the injunction to forbear from depriving another of them.[3] *Positive rights* such as the right to informed consent or the right to health care, on the other hand, merit consideration and modification within the context of other equally valued societal needs and opportunities, where trade-offs and questions of cost-effectiveness abound. To call such things rights may be understandable as an assertion of the primary value one tends to give them. It is also, I submit, symptomatic of a reticence to discuss the relative merits of different societal agendas and needs, and is part and parcel of the politics of confrontation, of the fervent insistence on single issues that plague our society and undermine a politics of rational debate and resolution. The Gordian knot that confronts us will not be severed by appeal to any such right, particularly the right to informed consent.

Respect for Patient Autonomy

Certain writers attempt to read a great deal into what the "respect for patient autonomy" requires of us, whatever the consequences and without regard for the effort required.[4] One case in point would be the insistence that mere permission to be treated is not enough, that "actual understanding" should routinely be assessed and if "substandard," then the informed consent should seek to enhance it. This work, however, finds no such richness in the idea of "respect for patient autonomy," at least in the sense that any rational being is necessarily bound to affirm such an obligation as operative. Rather, it sees such goods and values as variably at issue and more or less available from case to case and thus meriting varying degrees of pursuit. It will also be primarily concerned to address the autonomy interests of the common man, not those of members of the intellectual class. Such a preference will make us more willing to accept common preferences to trust matters to one's physician, to not be assaulted by the truth, or to respond to such matters with lack of interest.

Another basic bias of this work will be that a hard-nosed realism regarding the phenomenon of patient autonomy is absolutely necessary. There is too much of importance at stake here to proceed on the basis of sentimentality, theory-driven convictions, or untutored presumptions. One way to signal this bias is to concur with Daniel Callahan's concern that we may have bought the luxury of autonomy at too high a price (Callahan, 1984). That is, by presuming patient competence and ignoring or discounting its deficiencies, certain proponents of the "new ethos" may have undermined an equally vital need at the bedside—the physician who also embraces a commitment to beneficence for the sake of those rendered frail, vulnerable, and in need of assistance by the onslaught of illness.[5]

It should be noted that the preceding point constitutes that part of the message of this work that many in philosophy and the law will particularly wish to reject. In a number of forums in which I have presented some of the preceding argument, I have encountered two intertwined objections repeatedly. The first is that I disparage patients. The second is that I am providing confirmation of clinicians' skepticism.

Regarding the latter point, I do not believe that the pronouncements of a mere philosopher add any substance to common clinician views that are daily reconfirmed by experience. Some clinicians surely tend to overstate the problem, particularly when they launch into their "myth of informed consent" diatribe. My antidote to this problem, however, is not to attempt to ignore or argue away what is often obvious to the most casual observer. Rather, it is to accept such findings (hopefully without overstating what is actually the case) and then proceed to the more precarious enterprise of pursuing the goods and values that are no less at stake for being difficult to attain. As to the former point regarding disparaging patients, it seems that I am being charged with being "politically incorrect" by questioning the unaided cognitive and decision-making capacities of patients. To this I plead guilty. I prefer realism to wishful thinking that results only in cynically provided rituals and their sequelae: the abandonment of patients.

The Nature of the Argument of This Work

Our Gordian knot will thus not be severed in this work by appeal to any particular ethical theory, or primary right, or to "richer" extrapolations from the notion of respect for persons. Nor will sentimentality, political correctness, or questionable presumptions be allowed to make a case that the facts will not support. We will instead travel the much murkier and more difficult path where multiple consequences and possibilities must be evaluated, and the court at which we submit to judgment will proceed on the basis of numerous criteria, including the clarity and coherence of our formulations, as well as their applicability, realism, efficiency, and effectiveness. And whether the model "works" and is "cost-effective" will be a final court of appeal, regarding which a few basic considerations should now be arrayed.

THE BASIC STRUCTURE OF THE
MODEL ADVOCATED IN THIS WORK

To commit to the enterprise of seeking to resolve our "problem" of informed consent by providing an operational model involves identifying and making certain choices at the outset. As far as the clinical perspective goes, it will hardly receive an adequate response in our deliberations unless a thoroughgoing realism is adopted regarding the capacities and needs of patients. Equally, concern for the effective and efficient provision of informed consent must surely be operative, efforts thus connected to attainable goals, couched in formulations that are coherent and provide sufficient guidance to health care professionals. Referring back to the "sources" identified in the preceding chapters, progress can be made here in a relatively straightforward way.

The Need for a Standardized Basic Model

With all this talk about variables and spectrums, one might anticipate a very flexible, ad hoc model of informed consent will be offered in this work. This is not the case; there are a number of goods and values that must be provided for in any informed consent. Clearly some sort of basic disclosure must be provided in all cases, at least toward the enterprise of gaining a patient's authorization to proceed, and its character should be statable in clear terms. Even though patients' needs and capacities vary (as chapters 3 and 4 instruct us), we can expect neither the law nor society nor the majority of those writing in ethics to accept a totally flexible view resting completely on the physician's perception of the needs and opportunities at hand. Legal concerns that tend to require some degree of standardization of provision will further constrain us. Some across-the-board version of informed consent, however minimal or elaborate, must be offered.

Even if there were no legal or societal insistence on standardized informed consents, however, there are strong ethical and clinical reasons for articulating standard features that all should incorporate. Most basically, there are certain goods and values that should be pursued in every instance where an intervention is offered to a competent patient. The authorization of the patient to proceed should be gained, not just in some formal sense, or for legal purposes, but also toward creating the psychological reality that the patient has bought into the enterprise, has taken responsibility for it. The potential benefit of such an assumption of responsibility for patient compliance and cooperation should be apparent to clinicians, however much the cognitive bent of the scholarly literature has led to its not being given appropriate emphasis. Equally, though we will remain somewhat skeptical as to how much actual understanding patients typically attain, some fairly detailed rendition of the risks, benefits, and alternatives would at least address a negative sort of rule-out agenda. That is, such a presentation, however little actual detailed understanding it may produce, can still be valuable in that it would tend to identify the hesitant or ambivalent patient (or the patient who suddenly realizes that he is getting into much more than he anticipated). Again, it should be apparent that good medical management should seek to identify such problems up front rather than wait to deal with their sequelae. And we thus already have clinical and ethical agendas that call for significant content for informed consents for every medical intervention.

There are other important reasons for such standardization. (1) It is inequitable for different patients to receive markedly different informed consents for the same procedure simply because they are being treated by different physicians who happen to have different biases and agendas in this area. This is not to rule out the need for judgment calls concerning what is appropriate in a given instance, but certain standard disclosures and tactics are necessary with many procedures, and the profession should establish these. This book will not go to this level of specificity, but the model it will shortly offer will provide a general format and structure within which such specific content should be arrayed. (2) Absent any explicit or in-practice standard, student and resident physicians are not given any consistent direction regarding their responsibilities in a given situation, and the perception grows that the choices are arbitrary and personal. And given that we are speaking of the art of communicating with patients, with all that rides upon it, surely this part of their education should not be left to some inchoate process of osmosis at the bedside, or presented as if it were some add-on to medical care, the specific provision and form of which turns on one's personal preferences. The degree to which any of our previously identified goods and values are at stake or attainable in a given clinical situation will vary markedly. But the way in which a competent physician pursues such goods and values, when they *are* at stake, merits as structured and reflective a pursuit as any other intervention.

The need for a standardized model can also be demonstrated by making a philosophical point about the basic deficiency of the "ethical process" that the ethical theory of act-utilitarianism advocates. Some philosophers advance a view similar to the common clinician's contention that "every patient is unique" and use this to argue against a system of general, standardized rules. There are significant flaws to this position, however. We are creatures of habit, enhance our overall effectiveness by being such, and are prudent to be so as many situations (or patients) are not relevantly dissimilar. Put another way, we do not and need not reinvent the wheel every time we need one. Simple pragmatism calls for operational guidelines, or "standard operating procedures." These have the further advantage of being teachable to the neophyte, as well as being the ground for both establishing and honoring the expectations of those with whom we have congress. For informed consent as well, then, we need to fashion a detailed and ordered sense of what must minimally be provided in all cases, as to both the goals addressed and the tactics used.

A Heterogeneity of Needs and Possibilities

Beyond honoring the need for structure and regularity, we will equally be obliged to leave a place for flexible and discretionary responses to relevantly *dissimilar* variables as we move from case to case. Whatever minimum will be required, a place must also be allotted for the pursuit of additional goods and values that may be at stake in certain cases, however often or rarely. Such activities as the actual participation of patients in decision making and the enterprise of assessing the "actual understanding" of patients will be seen as not always necessary but sometimes essential, depending on the case at hand. Sometimes the inattentive patient will be acceptable, at other times intolerable. Equally, the degree that "actual understanding" in the patient is important, and merits some form of assessment as well as enhancement, will vary depending on the case at hand. Consider the situation of a patient with metastatic disease who presents with a bilateral infiltrate. Surely a good deal more needs to be discussed with this patient than simply the relative merits of various antibiotics—for example, whether he wants fully aggressive management if he decompensates further. Actual patient insight into the issues at hand in such a situation is much to be preferred and is likely to be absent without substantial assistance from the physician. To the autonomist who fears that patients' rights may evaporate in the fog of physician flexibility and discretion, I respond that such discretion is exercised anyway, the current "result" hardly suffices so there is little to evaporate, and one should await the formulation of what we will see as minimally necessary.

Informed Consent—Event or Process?

A basic point of contention about informed consent has been whether it should usually be offered as a discrete event or as some more flexible process extending over time. To the extent we are concerned to generate rules of thumb for the minimal provision of informed consent, a discrete, *event* model of informed consent is attractive. Certain agendas will always need to be pursued, such as gaining the patient's authorization, ruling him out for hesitation or ambivalence, or providing the previously stressed reassurance that comes from the physician's diagnosing the patient's problem and discussing what can be done about it. Such agendas should not be randomly embedded somewhere in the clinical interaction but rather should be given some specific, formal place, usually at the point where therapy is going to be initiated or modified. Equally, such a one-shot intervention has the advantage of signaling to the patient that a significant choice is at hand, rather than allowing such choices to be obscured or overlooked within some more free-flowing process.

Recognition of the further heterogeneity of needs and possibilities that informed consent may need to respond to in certain cases, however, tends to push us in the direction of some more flexible *process*—an ongoing enterprise where patient insight is developed and reassessed, and where less common needs are responded to when they become more important in individual cases. However much we may question the idea that detailed actual understanding by the patient is commonly needed, it can clearly be an important, at times paramount, need in certain instances.

To the preceding considerations, we should note some further virtues of a process model. (1) It recognizes that true, detailed insight by patients may well need time to build, allied to the anticipation of potential future problems or impending decisions, and with feedback and counseling after the fact. These are all part of the same enterprise, if informed consent is to attempt to accomplish what we might hope for from it. (2) Only by a process of ongoing assessment and exploration can patients and physicians truly come to a meeting of minds, a result that is particularly important in chronic illness, as well as when therapy involves long-term compliance issues. In this regard, it seems worth emphasizing that for the physician-patient relationship to have any real substance at all, such a process must occur, and informed consent, not just as an event but as an ongoing process of engagement and edification of each party as to the other's concerns, merits a large place in this. The aforementioned problem of the alienating medical assembly line, of "strangers taking care of strangers," can come to be as pathological a factor in certain situations as sepsis. (3) To the extent the case at hand calls for substantial "actual understanding" on the part of the patient, thus involving detailed assessment of it as well as efforts to enhance it, an ongoing process is required, as it would be in situations where more wide-ranging counseling of the patient regarding his situation and prospects are requisite. No one-shot event can be expected to have much success in pursuing such goals. (4) A process model recognizes that medical care is often spread over time with multiple decision points in the abstract, but where the more fundamental decision involves the ongoing acceptance of and participation in a complex therapeutic enterprise. A process model can verify and strengthen what an event model cannot.

Informed Consent as Both Process and Event

The response of this work to this seeming dichotomy will be to embrace the notion that informed consent has both event and process aspects, depending on the case, issues, and participants at hand. To opt for an essentially process approach would be to ignore the substantial advantages that an event model can offer. A mainly static "event" model, for its part, would fail to provide for the many nuances and variables that we have repeatedly identified.

To anticipate, the model offered in the remainder of this work will involve an event model of informed consent with regard to the highlighting of basic, discrete choices, the gaining of permission from the patient, and the articulation of what seems minimally necessary in all cases. The process aspect will receive concurrent consideration here, particularly in that we need to clarify what opportunities and tactics exist in situations where one needs to go beyond some minimal informed consent event. Such will be the case when further counseling is needed, long-term compliance must be stimulated, or simply, the relationship between physician and patient must be further developed by giving it real content and mutuality.

However crucial the process aspect of informed consent is in particular cases, however, our model will incorporate a strong bias toward accomplishing most of the goals of informed consent in most cases within the framework of discrete informed consent events. This is, I submit, the format where we should place our money in the vast majority of cases. This is so for a number of reasons. (1) Again, such an event tends to emphasize the fact of choice and need for attention to the issues at hand, and these factors would tend to be submerged in a more free-flowing process. Such an activity is also more readily documented, as well as standardized both as a generic model and with

reference to particular interventions. (2) Much of the further assessment, clarification, and counseling that certain thinkers tend to see as
requiring a process sort of approach are, as the first part of chapter 4
suggests, often not necessary. Often the choice at hand is legitimately
seen by both patient and physician as clearly indicated and not meriting any further discussion or reflection. So the sorts of goals that especially call for a process model are often not at issue. (3) It equally
seems, in other cases, that such further discussion, assessment, and
counseling are essential to the discrete choice itself and should not be
left to a process deferred to another time. Here one might think of the
insertion of a central line for diagnostic and therapeutic purposes in a
patient with an exacerbation of severe chronic obstructive pulmonary
disease. To simply discuss the immediate pros and cons of the central
line without placing this act within the context of an overall aggressive course of management is hardly an adequate representation of the
choice at hand, nor does it identify the issues that need to be considered. To buy into the central line is, by implication, to buy into a great
deal more, especially an aggressive orientation to the management of
a disease that may only result in more suffering without rectifying
even the immediate problem. It is the latter that the patient might particularly want and need to reflect on. (4) It should be clear that the regular provision of discrete informed consent events is not only one way
in which a process model would be conducted—its "bits and pieces,"
as it were—but would provide the necessary foundation for any such
further process, especially one that pursues such needs as coping and
adaptation to chronic disease, or the sort of existential reflection that a
terminal illness calls for. One of my most basic perceptions as an ethics
consultant is that many of the problems and disputes between physicians and patients, especially over aggressive treatment, are caused
primarily by the absence of any ongoing attempt to educate and counsel the patient beforehand. It is high time that the medical profession
recognize that trying to get hypoxic patients to decide whether they
want intubation at crisis time is just bad practice. No one should be
comfortable with whatever answer is given at such a juncture, and it is
simply an abuse of the patient's trust not to have anticipated what are
often quite foreseeable scenarios and give the patient time and assistance to make such a decision at his leisure. The etiology here lies, at
best, in a false compassion that mainly protects the clinician from
disagreeable conversations, and often at the price of substantial harm
and suffering to the patient down the line. Katz's "silent world of

doctor and patient" can thus become a profoundly pathological world, and discrete informed consent events, however leavened by an ensuing process, can provide much of the needed "therapeutic" response to this silence.

To emphasize the primacy of informed consent events in our account is not to depreciate the value of the surrounding process. An overall atmosphere of trust, candor, information provision, assessment, and feedback is surely essential to the effectiveness and success of any physician-patient encounter. To treat a patient as a child to be managed, where passivity is accepted if not extolled, stacks the deck against the chance that when a discrete decision is at hand the patient will somehow rise to the occasion. Any discrete informed consent event should thus be more broadly construed as potentially involving a more wide-ranging, give-and-take discussion, either when the patient somehow signals the need for it, or when the physician does. We may be emphasizing an event model here, but it is not to be a static ritual as presently is par for the course.

Our next three chapters will primarily focus on the event aspect of our operational model of informed consent. Our tactic will be to return to the categories that were articulated by the law at the outset of this discussion—the nature of competence, the considerations affecting what will be disclosed to the patient and in what form, and the issues raised when we consider not only whether the patient understands what is going on but the considerations affecting the patient's evaluation and consent to (or refusal of) the data and recommendations thus provided. As with the law, we will also pause to reflect on possible exceptions to the rule of providing informed consent—for example, in emergencies or when patients voluntarily waive informed consent.

NOTES

1. There are numerous introductory chapters to editions of bioethics articles that offer adequate short introductions to ethics and basic terminology. To the person particularly interested in such an introduction, I would recommend Beauchamp and Childress (1989).

2. See, for example, Engelhardt (1986), pp. 104–56.

3. Even such basic rights are sometimes alternatively treated as "justified claims." I will not quarrel with this. My basic point would still be that

such basic "rights" or "justified claims" must still be sharply differentiated from the many other "claims" that are the stuff of political trade-offs and compromise, the former being essential to any moral and just society.

4. Regarding what I consider to be an especially "overcooked" treatment of the requirements of respect for patient autonomy, see my review of Richard Zaner's *Ethics and the Clinical Encounter* in Wear (1987).

5. See Jackson and Youngner (1979) for the classic article that details just such an undermining—clinicians too quickly accepting patient directives as legitimate. They found, for example, that patient consents to DNR orders were impeached when, on further investigation, such factors as clinically treatable depression and significant patient misconceptions about their situation and prospects were found to be in the background.

6

The Informed Consent Event

In order to fashion a synthesis of the various agendas and perspectives that weigh upon us, we have elected to give primacy to an informed consent event in our account, however much it may need to be augmented by a surrounding process. The informed consent event has three distinct stages, each aimed at quite different though complementary goals: (1) the *comprehensive disclosure* stage, which will roughly approximate the detailed presentation of risks, benefits, and alternatives of a given intervention required by American law but will be aimed at more modest goals, such as providing the patient the opportunity to rule in or out regarding hesitancy, ambivalence, or misconceptions; (2) the *core disclosure* stage, which will attempt to counter the information-overload tendency of the first stage and give patients something relatively simple and structured that they might minimally react to and evaluate—namely, the essential choice at hand; and (3) the *assessment, clarification, and patient choice* stage, which will be the only necessarily interactive part of the informed consent event (unless the patient spontaneously chooses this mode at any other point), and which will key to the specific patient's level of understanding and other concerns. This stage will proceed by probing into the patient's understanding of the information provided in the preceding two stages and will respond to this with appropriate clarification of the patient's developing sense of the issues at hand.

As we proceed through each of the three stages, four basic issues will repeatedly face us. (1) What are the explicit, intended goals of each stage? (2) What specific content should each stage have? (3) How will this content be arrayed so as to be maximally accessible to the patient? Much more than a shopping list is required to pursue the goals we have identified. (4) What sort of variables may modify the conduct of each stage, either as part of the discrete event, or toward triggering a longer process of education and counseling?

STAGE I: THE COMPREHENSIVE DISCLOSURE

For those clinicians who practice in areas where the law on informed consent has evolved to the level portrayed in chapter 1, the primary purpose of the "comprehensive disclosure" stage might be regarded as no more than insurance against a malpractice suit. I will presume to suggest that this stage may well satisfy this legal agenda, where it is operative, especially by its comprehensive detail. But, as previously stressed, clinicians should consult legal counsel in their particular jurisdiction on such matters.

Turning to clinical and ethical considerations, the major goals of this stage are (1) to provide the grounds for an adequate rule-out of hesitancy, ambivalence, and misconceptions on the patient's part; (2) to provide a first step toward developing a mature physician-patient relationship, as well as, by the force of its detail, possibly stimulating the common, inattentive patient to recognize that serious matters are at hand and respond with a heightened level of attentiveness; and (3) to motivate a patient to assume personal responsibility for a given decision, which requires some degree of explicit content regarding what the intervention amounts to. The trust at the core of the physician-patient relationship might well be undermined if the patient subsequently suffers a known, relatively common risk of an intervention that the clinician did not even mention up front.

The reader should note that we are not listing the goal of actual understanding among our agendas at this stage. Detailed presentation of information does not directly produce a mature, comprehensive understanding, however much some patients may be able to parrot back a fairly comprehensive list. Some patients will grasp this presentation in a comprehensive fashion, and we can hope for this; but it will not be an expected result of this stage.

A tactical note is also in order: at any point or stage in any process of communication with a patient one may well need to move from a monologue to something more interactive. This first comprehensive disclosure stage might well proceed throughout on a monologue basis, absent some sort of rule-in indication from the patient. If the rule-out agenda is going to have some potential to be effective, however, it must cue to factors beyond the explicit questions of the patient. Body language and facial expressions can be quite revealing, as can oral indicators such as the pitch and tone of the patient's voice. They may well be the only signs of a problem that merits response.

One may, of course, ask patients if they have questions at any juncture, but such generic questioning seems to have a low yield.

One might also specifically request, at certain points, that the patient repeat what he has just heard, the clinician then responding to the patient's statements to the extent they lack detail or involve misconceptions. Such a potentially time-consuming tactic could be used at any juncture, but, given the typical time constraints, it need not be used in this stage unless there is a rule-in indication from the patient. The goal of the informed consent event, as previously articulated, is *not* actual understanding by the patient at this level of detail and complexity. Such a goal will be explicitly pursued in the second and third stages of the informed consent event, and it will later be suggested that at least a generic actual understanding is a major goal with any competent patient during the overall *process* of treatment and communication. But barring any specific indication, such a tactic is not advocated as a necessary part of this first stage for reasons of efficiency as well as not forcing a patient to perform in ways he does not wish.

Turning to the specific structure and content of the "comprehensive disclosure" stage, we will follow the law's guidance regarding the specific types of information that any informed consent should incorporate. These are, in sum, the patient's overall medical condition, the specific problem for which treatment is being recommended, the treatment recommended with its attendant benefits and risks, any alternative modalities, and the prognosis without treatment.

The Broader Context of the Decision at Hand

My own experience, and that of colleagues I have questioned, is that there is a strong tendency by physicians to focus on the immediate issues and options at hand in pursuing informed consent, with little or no attempt to locate this discussion within the broader context of the patient's medical history or his overall situation and prospects. This is not surprising, even when the practitioner is not cynical about informed consent, as the immediate aim of this "intervention"— informed consent—is to get the patient's authorization to proceed with treatment.

Such an approach may well be the most efficient way to reach this immediate goal, but it is also the best way of losing the battle regarding our other agendas at the outset. One hardly needs to appeal to some theory of understanding or communication to hold that such agendas are pursued in a meaningful way only by attaching the bits and pieces of disclosure to some more general framework that aids understanding, interpretation, and memory. We will thus depart from the usual emphasis on the content of disclosure per se by being equally concerned, in this section and throughout, with the manner in which any detail is communicated and arrayed.

For many patients, such a general framework will involve no more than that they are otherwise healthy, and the presenting problem is some sort of acute, discrete problem that may well be completely and permanently reversible, such as gall bladder removal in an otherwise healthy patient suffering from stone. In others, the problem may be partially the result of patient behaviors that should be identified as self-destructive, like the role of smoking in chronic bronchitis. But for many other patients, there is a specific and detailed context within which treatment will occur and specific interventions will be offered. The patient with an advanced carcinoma needs to be thinking about much more than immediate treatment options when hypercalcemia occurs. This may well be an end-stage phenomenon that needs to be appreciated as such, as well as considered as offering a potentially much more palatable exit than what may come after it (e.g., metastases to bone). Similarly, the patient with advanced cirrhosis who has started to bleed and the post–MI patient with recurrent shortness of breath have specific contexts within which to appreciate and evaluate any proposed intervention.

The point, however, is not primarily to provide for the possibility of treatment refusal. Rather, it is to begin with some individualized expression of the patient's past medical history and the identification of ways in which it may have caused or contributed to the problem at hand. In short, the patient should be instructed as to who he is from an overall medical point of view, thus providing a framework within which the patient can get a sense of his more immediate problems and options. Clearly such a basic context will vary from the very simple to the quite detailed and complex.

As mentioned, my own sense is that this sort of framework is often not provided. Further, this framework is especially valuable as a communication aid, because patients often seem to have at least idiosyncratic, if not misconceived or false, conceptions at this level. Self-destructive behaviors like drinking, smoking, and obesity are often not appreciated as such. Just as often, the potentially chronic or even terminal quality of a given generic illness is not well perceived. In part such flaws are often patient-generated, from denial, for example, or an unwillingness to accept responsibility. Experience also counsels, I submit, that one should *not* assume that the patient's previous physician has made a sufficient effort to bring the patient to insight about his situation and prospects. These are often difficult, uncomfortable discussions for all concerned. Many physicians, as well as patients, still respond to such tasks with avoidance behavior. Hence our first rule-out regards whether the patient has an adequate understanding of himself as a patient with a history, and whether he has other collateral or contributory problems.

Diagnosis

Having provided the "context" of a given intervention, one should be careful to separate the specific problem to be addressed from this background. That a given intervention, the one for which consent is being sought, responds to only one of a number of problems should be clearly indicated to the patient. Labeling also seems to help. Among other things, patients seem to intuitively understand that making a specific diagnosis is often more than half the battle and often indicates a definite therapeutic response. Such labeling provides reassurance, as well as tends to diminish what may have been a quite gnawing uncertainty. Diagnostic labels alone are, however, insufficient at this stage and should be explicated by reference to the signs and symptoms the patient is presenting. What, in effect, does this diagnosis come to, experientially and functionally, for this particular patient?[1]

Prognosis without Treatment

The structure of a given informed consent may well vary given the situation at hand, but it would seem, as a rule of thumb, that this item is best presented prior to the specific therapeutic recommendation. This is so as one already will have provided both the general and specific context for intervention. The prognosis without treatment might best be seen as closely allied to the diagnosis in the sense that it is what the problem amounts to in the absence of any therapeutic response. It is also another valuable "framework" for understanding in that it provides the natural history of the disease that the subsequent recommended therapy will more or less cure, ameliorate, or palliate.

    The prognosis without treatment also seems to merit mention early on as it signals what is at least abstractly true for any therapeutic situation—that there is always the choice of no further treatment at all. This is not to say that either the patient or the physician will see the choice of no therapy in a given situation as even remotely reasonable.[2] But it is the backdrop against which the subsequent rendition of the benefits and risks of a recommended intervention should be minimally evaluated. In the usual case, this will amount to no more than a listing of all the reasons why it would be unwise for the patient to just grin and bear it. But it does also have the merit of emphasizing the fact that a choice is always abstractly present. To the extent that some patients do make this choice for no therapy in the situation at hand (e.g., in the case of advanced metastatic disease), this fact should also be emphasized. In sum, the physician alerts the patient that he may well wish to consider not having any therapy at all, and the subsequent offer of a therapeutic response is thus announced as something other than the obvious and necessary course to take.

The Recommended Treatment with Attendant Risks and Benefits

This is the heart of any informed consent. As a practical matter, it often makes up the entire conversation, with little reference given to the previous "contexts" or to alternative modalities. It also often seems to be offered more as a sales pitch than a neutral presentation of pros and cons. There are often, of course, sufficient grounds for a physician to make a recommendation to a patient, and in such cases the real task lies in avoiding a biased sort of sales pitch in favor of an honest rendition of the pros and cons of what the physician tends to prefer.

Our previous discussions also suggest that the presentation of a specific recommendation will *not* be appropriate in certain cases. For one thing, profound and personal choices may be in the offing, and these preclude any firm recommendation from the clinician, at least prior to substantial discussion with the patient (e.g., in newly diagnosed metastatic disease). In such a case, this section would need to be converted into a more complex presentation of alternatives with no one option recommended. A more subtle situation may also be at hand where the clinician has a preference but recognizes that there are real grounds for the patient to choose an alternative modality. That such grounds exist is apparent simply from the fact that similarly situated patients have been known to make different choices. In such an instance, an up-front recommendation by the physician may be counterproductive.

Recommendations by the physician may also be seen as having broader counterproductive tendencies. As Haavi Morreim has suggested:

> I have serious reservations about the scenario in which the physician automatically presumes that he must center his disclosure around a recommendation. That can place the patient in a very difficult position if he genuinely wants to talk more about alternatives. Many patients do not want to appear contrary, or to bear the burden of refusing, objecting, demanding, or engaging in other negative behaviors. In other words, in a model that has the physician automatically present the information in the form of a recommendation, the patient who wants to look seriously at his choices is placed in a socially awkward position.[3]

At this juncture, I will proceed as though a recommendation can be legitimately offered by the clinician. Part of my response to Professor Morreim's concern will come in the form of the ensuing section's reflection on the various ways that the "alternative treatment" disclosure can be pursued. A second response is that she has identified one of the basic variables that any informed consent event must assess. It may be advisable, for example, to respond to patient hesitancy or ambivalence by at least initially withholding a recommendation that might serve to only temporarily submerge such factors. Suffice it to say, at this juncture, that clinicians often emerge from their workup of a patient with a clear therapeutic preference, see no sense in which an alternative modality is legitimate, and are simply responding to the patient's desire for a specific recommendation. There are other ways to stimulate patients to make their subjective concerns known without forcing the clinician to hold back on giving his patient the benefit of his knowledge and experience in situations where the physician feels they have clear implications. The second and third stages of this model aim primarily at such interaction.

Identifying the Potential Benefits of a Given Intervention

We should thus say that an informed consent should seek to avoid the "sales pitch" mode, while at the same time usually offering the recommendation the patient seeks, assuming that a basic commonality of values is likely. This approach has some clear corollaries. (1) Benefits should be stated in functional terms, not in terms of biochemical or occult anomalies. One's language should key to the signs and symptoms that the patient presents. (2) Given that the most ideal benefit would be full, instantaneous, painless, inexpensive, convenient, and permanent cure, the ways in which the results of the recommended intervention may fall short of this ideal should also be stressed. Such a statement of the predictable or possible ways that the proposed intervention may fall short of this ideal may well be the most effective and appropriate way to package this information. In sum, the limitations of the intervention must be explicated, whether these regard the sense of a cure as being only partial, with some chronic residue, or that cure will take time, perhaps being dependent on later rehabilitative efforts, or that there might well be a recurrence even if the problem is removed for a time. A patient being treated for a stroke would be an obvious example of someone who needs to understand that such limitations of treatment are definitely present. (3) Such limitations should also key to the two previous contexts of the patient's overall medical situation as well as the specific problem that is being addressed. The specific problem (e.g., shortness of breath from pneumonia) might well be totally resolved while contributory chronic illness (e.g., obstructive pulmonary disease) remains unaffected, and recurrence of the present problem, or new ones, predictable or possible. In sum, any statement of benefits should be offered hand in hand with a sense of their limitations.

Identifying Risks and Potential Complications

Perhaps the hardest thing for physicians to do is give an accurate rendition of the risk and complication profile of a given intervention. Even when they believe in the enterprise of seeking informed consent, this part of it clearly goes against the grain in various ways. (1) It has its own risks in the sense of potentially creating a "nocebo" effect where mentioned risks or complications tend to occur at a higher rate or greater intensity. The classic instance here is when one mentions the potential side effect of impotence of a certain drug. Not only does the psychogenic component of impotence give such a nocebo effect room to operate, but removal of the drug in response to resultant impotence may well not remove the complication. To those committed to the best interests of the patient, such considerations are disconcerting. (2) We must remember that whatever goals we ascribe to the informed consent event, the psychological reality of it for the physician is that, having gone through a process of testing, assessment, and diagnosis, he is now, usually and primarily, offering the patient a recommendation as to how to proceed. Mention of the downsides of the proposal is thus contrary to the primary enterprise. (3) The specification of risks and complications by the physician, on a personal level, will probably arise in large part not just from a literature search, or formal education, but from the physician's own experience with those patients for whom the recommended therapy went awry, in certain cases disastrously or lethally. To expect physicians to retail risks and complications, then, is to request that they, in a certain sense, function in a superhuman way in that they must act contrary to their primary aim of gaining consent, be unaffected by what may be searing past experience, and do something that may itself adversely affect the success of the intervention. And all this with a patient who probably has expressed no more than a desire for treatment and humane care.

The first point regarding risk disclosure, then, is that physicians should approach it with an explicit sense that they are going against their own grain in various ways and need to be on guard that this does not keep them from adequately accomplishing the legitimate, even if disconcerting and counterproductive, tasks at hand. What are the legitimate tasks at hand, particularly at this stage of the "comprehensive disclosure"?

It is, first of all, to list those ways in which the treatment, whether it succeeds in its primary purposes or not, may well have its own negative aspects. Some factors may simply go with the turf—significant pain after an open heart operation, nausea and lethargy from certain medications, or a long convalescence, bed-bound or not. Others will be probabilities or possibilities only, and part of the task will be to divide these up into (1) major risks or complications that bear individual identification, with attendant statistics, and (2) lesser ones that might instead be noted together with their rate of occurrence expressed for the group as a whole, not individually.

And how do we identify major and more minor risks, both per se and within the context of the much more numerous risks to which most interventions are theoretically liable? A few caveats may be offered that cannot provide precise guidance in individual cases but seem to be the most one can say. (1) One direct way to identify major risks will be simply on the basis of what the physician will be most worried about as he proceeds and for which he will be particularly concerned to monitor. The physician might particularly key to any downside of a given intervention that gives pause when he is considering a certain recommendation. (2) Past experience with patients should be helpful, keying to what they were most disconcerted by, whether it was resultant pain, a long hospital stay, or disorientation. It should be remembered that we are not just providing abstract grounds for refusal by means of such information, which may well not even be a remote possibility. We are also providing the downsides of the course of treatment, the nature of the price the patient may be forced to pay. It would seem that there is no better way to destroy the physician-patient relationship than to provide the patient with a false and sugar-coated sense of what he is about to undergo, the risks he is about to run. (3) The principle of "when in doubt, mention it" seems to have some legitimacy, particularly as the further stages of the informed consent event will not function under such a standard and will have the goal of directing the patient to the essentials of the choice at hand, beyond all the only potentially significant detail. (4) One often finds legal writings mentioning that "commonly known" risks of an intervention need not be mentioned. As we have already noted, however, clinical experience suggests that one cannot assume that a given patient in fact is aware of what is "commonly known," and that if a risk is in fact commonly known it is probably because it has true significance and, thus, the law aside, candor and credibility with the patient dictate that this exception to disclosure not be utilized.

Is this all that can be said by way of guidance regarding what to disclose? It appears that we are still coming up with rather thin gruel, and doing little better than the legal guidance that we criticized so sharply earlier. Further assistance may be gained here by reflecting on the suggestion by Appelbaum, Lidz, and Meisel that risks have four primary aspects—nature, magnitude, percentage of occurrence, and immanence (Appelbaum et al., 1987, p. 51). The *nature* of a given risk should primarily be stated in terms of signs and symptoms that would be involved for the patient, however much one refers to more occult anomalies by way of explanation. Equally, an essential part of the nature of a given risk will reside in the ways in which it may lead to other problems, adversely affect the treatment or convalescence, or call for further interventions with risks and complications of their own. The *magnitude* of a given risk, for its part, is a function of its abstract significance should it occur, the ways in which it might adversely affect treatment and convalescence, involve further interventions, and basically assault the quality of life, well-being, and functioning of the patient. The *percentage of occurrence* and *immanence* move the consideration from that of abstract threat to real possibility.

Again, I believe the standard of practice leaves something to be desired. Along with mainly providing a list of risks and complications, physicians usually seem to key to the abstract aspect of magnitude here in selecting for disclosure. In this regard, "four alarm" risks such as death, brain damage, and paralysis often get emphasized even if they are very unlikely although occasional risks of a given intervention. But it seems clear that one has the option of identifying such rare complications within a group listing of minor risks, as opposed to giving them independent emphasis and specification, particularly beyond what they merit.

As to which risks merit individual specification and emphasis, the selection should turn on an *integral* consideration of *magnitude* and *percentage* of occurrence. The issue of when a given risk becomes "major," because either one of these two aspects is substantial or both are significantly high, must key to professional practice, the physician's sense of what patients seem to find particularly significant, and those things that cause the physician to pause or think twice about offering the intervention in question. Finally, given that the core disclosure stage will tend to focus the patient more toward the essentials and the bottom line, elevation of a particular risk from a minor one that will be listed within a group, to a major, individually specified one should be guided by the principle: "When in doubt, elevate it to a major risk."

A further type of risk deserves mention, as it appears that it often does not receive the emphasis it merits. Beyond the various discrete risks of an intervention per se, there are negative aspects of the overall nature and environment of treatment that may well be quite significant. One such factor lies in the act of hospitalization itself, where sick, often frail people are inserted into a milieu where resistant organisms are present in abundance, and much more than they bargained for may well occur. I am thinking specifically of a hospital admission to provide intravenous antibiotics for a patient with an otherwise recalcitrant infection. Clearly such admissions often lead to further problems, particularly in the frail elderly, and hindsight at least seems to dictate that one might well have thought twice about such a course of action (Office of Technology Assessment, 1987, pp. 333–447).

Another such broader negative aspect involves the impact on a patient's overall life of a given course of treatment, not so much in the sense of medical risks and complications, but in inconvenience and extra expense. A good example is that of chronic renal dialysis, where the treatment often takes up three afternoons a week, not to mention the expense and inconvenience of getting to these sessions. The fact that a significant number of patients later opt for renal transplant, even in the face of its higher mortality and morbidity, seems to be in large part traceable to such factors and thus signals information that merits mention and emphasis up front—*not* that such considerations dictate that a physician should necessarily give much more place to the alternative of transplantation at the start of chronic renal failure. It may well be that the less "risky" avenue of dialysis should be tried first toward seeing how the patient will tolerate it. But such considerations do suggest that we are also speaking of a major downside of a treatment here and thus should stress it as such.

It should finally be emphasized that the discussion of risks and benefits here will usually come as part of a broader presentation that offers the patient a specific recommendation of how to proceed. Given this, the discussion of risks should not simply take on the aspect of some discrete discussion within the informed consent event but should also have an interrelative aspect in two senses: the risks and complications should be directly portrayed and evaluated with reference to (1) the counterbalancing benefits of the proposed intervention, and (2) the risks, complications, and overall negative sequelae of nontreatment. As at any juncture, this could well deteriorate into a sales pitch. The trick is to make the case for the proposed intervention to the patient without biasing the presentation in an inappropriate way. And here, as at other junctures of the informed consent event, heightened insight and appreciation by the patient might well be gained by concluding this part of the presentation with a clear statement why the physician feels that the aforementioned risks and potential complications are worth being exposed to for the sake of the treatment recommended and relative to the result if such treatment is not provided. The informed consent event should repeatedly, then, recapitulate and tie into its early stages.

Our response to the thorny problem of what to disclose to the patient regarding the risks of a given treatment should, in effect, be appreciated as embracing the "hyperinforming" mode that we earlier sharply criticized in the law (or at least what many clinicians perceive as legally required). We have suggested that when in doubt as to the significance of a given risk, one should mention it, as well as give it individual emphasis, if one is unsure as to how significant it is. Such loquaciousness is not recommended with any belief that the patient will grasp such detail in any comprehensive or integrated fashion. Recall, for example, that Morgan and Schwab's study found that only 4 percent of patients recalled more than two out of five disclosed risks (Morgan and Schwab, 1986).

Actual understanding and retention of information are not the goals of this stage. One of our most basic aims in this first stage is to pursue a credible rule-out of hesitancy and ambivalence on the patient's part. *The wealth of detail allowed and encouraged in this stage, which will be particularly substantial in the area of risk disclosure, might thus be best appreciated as a sort of informational "stress test" for patients.* As to the hyperinforming criticism we made of the law, the response is that by providing better contexts and integration of these materials, by separating out more and less substantial risks, the latter presented in group form with an overall, not individual rate of occurrence, we hope somewhat to counter the information-overload problem. But the most basic response to this problem is contained in the second and third stages of the informed consent event, where such detail is absent from a more essential statement of the choice at hand and the patient's understanding, at such a more basic level of detail, is then assessed and responded to as needed.

Specification of Alternative Treatments

The final separate category of disclosure concerns other ways in which an illness might be treated as opposed to the intervention being recommended. On the one hand, this area has clearly become one of intense societal concern, whether we are talking generically about the issue of unnecessary surgery or about specific situations where alternative modalities may well be more attractive, even if not as effective, to a given patient, as, for example, the option of lumpectomy versus radical mastectomy for breast cancer. On the other hand, it seems accurate to say that there often is a clear, primary course of action, both from the physician's and the average patient's point of view, and extended discussions of individual alternatives might well have no other effect than to distract the patient from his primary task—understanding and evaluating the treatment being recommended.

There is actually a spectrum of choices regarding the presentation of alternatives. One extreme of this spectrum arises in the situation where there is no extant alternative and the choice is between the recommended treatment and no treatment at all. The opposite extreme occurs when, as anticipated, the physician may not even be able to legitimately offer a recommendation because the choice between two or more alternatives involves quite personal and profound values and issues to which only the patient can meaningfully speak. We should briefly canvass the types of scenarios in this spectrum.

Clear Treatment of Choice with No Alternatives

In such cases, only the alternative of no therapeutic response at all needs to be mentioned, and this, as noted, may well be only a theoretical choice that does not merit being taken seriously unless the patient insists. We must recognize that some informed consents will not be a matter of emphasizing a real choice for the patient, but will instead be intended to educate him about the only treatment available and solicit his authorization to proceed.

Clear Treatment of Choice with Alternatives Only from a Technical or Professional Point of View

The issue here concerns choices from among various modalities. These selections require expert judgment and experience and thus do not merit mention as they would require a fund of knowledge by patients that they neither do nor could possess—for example, choices between different drug regimens and different technical aspects of a surgical intervention. The decision not to mention such options should be based, however, not on the technical character of the differences but instead upon the fact that the risk-benefit profiles of such choices are essentially similar.

Alternative Modalities Exist, but the Physician Could Not Conscientiously Offer Them

These include modalities that in the abstract are sometimes offered for a given illness but are not reasonable alternatives given the patient's specific situation. The point of this presentation would be for the physician to mention such "options" and state clearly why he does not believe they are feasible. An example might be radiation for a discrete bowel tumor where surgical resection is the standard of practice and radiation considered substandard care or even malpractice. With all due respect for patient autonomy, physicians should not be forced to provide therapy that they consider inappropriate. But again, whether a given treatment is inappropriate should be determined by its technical aspects, not by more value-charged aspects where knowledgeable patients might choose differently. The aim in such situations is to rule out certain interventions that, though they are sometimes utilized in patients who, abstractly, have the same problem, are not seen as legitimate for the specific patient at hand.

Alternative Therapies Exist and Have Some Merit, but the Physician Feels the Recommended Treatment Has Substantial Advantages

This will often be the case in the informed consent situation, and the idea is not just that such alternatives should be described but that the physician should make clear, concurrently, why he considers them less attractive or appropriate. In effect, this part of the disclosure would be the negative side of the process of recommendation in that it identifies specific alternatives and makes clear why they are less worthy than the proposed course of action.

Alternative Modalities Exist, and One of Them May Well Be Preferred by the Patient, but the Physician Still Has a Marked Preference

The idea here is that the physician may still be offering the patient a recommendation, but he also recognizes that reasonable people might well choose one of the alternatives. That such a possibility exists may be suggested by the fact that similarly situated patients choose differently. It may also arise because the physician recognizes grounds for hesitancy in himself. This is the type of situation where the physician should be especially concerned to signal to the patient that there is some real choice at hand and make that choice clear to the patient. I am mainly thinking of situations where either two therapeutic options are similarly effective but involve different risk and complication pictures, or even if one is more effective, it also comes with a higher rate of morbidity or mortality, such as dialysis or transplant for chronic renal failure. That the physician still has a recommendation to offer in such a situation may well turn on no more than what he is used to providing, or what he would want if he were in the patient's shoes. Such weak grounds do not preclude giving a recommendation. We may well be in a situation where clinical insight and judgment, as well as the personal experience of the physician, have a good deal to say, and the patient should not be deprived of such counsel. But the other half of the task will be to advise the patient of the nontechnical, more conjectural nature of the grounds for the recommendation.

No Recommendation Can Legitimately Be Given, as the Alternatives Are Equally Appropriate and Reasonable

This category will definitely go against the grain of most physicians and patients, the former being used to giving recommendations, the latter expecting them. As previously discussed, however, there are clearly situations where the patient faces choices that are eminently personal and profound, and informed consent should be particularly aimed at helping the patient to see this. A paradigm situation would be a patient with a recurrent carcinoma where aggressive treatment has some efficacy, but might well do no more than produce added suffering and destroy what remaining good time he otherwise has left. There are many situations where varying rates of effectiveness of different treatments, and varying degrees of mortality and morbidity, can make the choice between two options very much six of one and a half-dozen of the other, with no objective grounds for choosing one over the other. For example, the ongoing argument over the appropriateness of medical or surgical management of certain forms of cardiac disease, where the dispute turns on different evaluations of the varying morbidity and mortality of the two options, is a good indication that more subjective judgments are at the heart of the dispute. It seems inappropriate that a given patient will receive one treatment as opposed to another merely because he is sitting in front of a surgeon rather than an internist.

The physician, in sum, must recognize when he is making nontechnical, value-laden judgments that patients might well evaluate differently. This is not to embrace the extreme view that such a discrepancy may often be present and needs to be pursued. As already suggested, physicians and patients generally do share basic values and beliefs, at least those relevant to the medical decisions at hand. *They are often not, in any interesting sense, moral strangers.* The point is that this last category insists that physicians should honestly announce to their patients that the choice at hand involves subjective, value-laden elements, and might well be seen differently by the patient if he is apprised of them.

A final point regarding the specification of alternative therapies is in order. We committed ourselves earlier to pack as much into the informed consent event as possible, avoiding relegating pertinent matters to some surrounding process. We also suggested that the informed consent event might well become quite complex and need to be quite flexible at certain junctures. One way to appreciate the point at which the informed consent event would be obliged to be more complex and flexible is by recognizing the need for this as alternative therapies become more credible. This means that real choices are present and should be discussed. It also means that the tendency of the patient to wait for the punchline probably ought to be challenged and further discussion ensue. Particularly when we get to the situation where profound and personal issues are at stake, where no clear recommendation can be offered, the typical informed consent monologue would need to give way to a true dialogue, even in the face of patient reticence.[4]

Thus ends our discussion of the first comprehensive disclosure stage of the informed consent event. Depending on the patient's situation and prospects, this stage may be quite simple and brief, as when ampicillin-sensitive pneumonia is diagnosed, or quite complex and lengthy, at all points, as in a discussion of metastatic disease. As noted, the goals of this stage will usually be more modest and negative, in the sense that we are giving the patient the *opportunity* to gain a full understanding of his situation and prospects, as well as rule himself in or out as to hesitancy, ambivalence, misconceptions, or a desire for more information or discussion. We do not, for reasons already outlined, bring any great optimism to this stage regarding most patients' ability or desire to gain a fully detailed or integrated and reflective grasp of this material. Greater expectations in this regard will, however, be brought to our second stage, core disclosure, to which we now turn.

STAGE II: THE CORE DISCLOSURE

As with the first stage, the second, core disclosure, stage[5] may well be fairly lengthy and complex in some cases, particularly where more or less equally attractive alternative modalities are present, or where profound and personal choices must be faced. But generally the second stage will be much simpler than its predecessor. The basic goal of this stage is to present the essentials of the choice at hand to the patient in an approachable and palatable fashion. This choice will often involve no more than asking the patient to choose to agree with the treatment recommended by the physician when, as anticipated, no reasonable alternative is seen to exist, and the option of nontreatment is accurately portrayed as unattractive. At the other extreme, the patient may be asked to engage in a profoundly personal assessment of alternative modalities, as well as to consider the nontreatment option. As already noted, there is a wide spectrum of the sense of choice here, and it is this actual, specific choice that the physician should now emphasize, absent much of the potentially stultifying detail. The aim of this stage should thus be seen as keying to the activity of choice, not the presentation of information, the latter already having been provided in detail. The nature of such a presentation, particularly in the sense of the perspective it will offer, has been previously addressed by another thinker, the physician-philosopher Howard Brody, and a review of his formulation will advance the search for our own.

The Transparency Model of Howard Brody

Sharing many of the same concerns that we have previously struggled with, Howard Brody proposed a "transparency" model of informed consent as a solution (Brody, 1989). Though Brody offered his model with specific reference to primary care situations, it might be proposed for all informed consent situations. And, as will now be seen, it might be particularly attractive to practicing physicians.

The essential point of Brody's model is that, instead of providing the usual complex and content-filled informed consents, physicians avoid such potentially self-stultifying detail in favor of "making transparent" to the patient why they prefer and are recommending a given therapy. Such a presentation might well mention a number of risks, or even discuss an alternative modality, not for the wider informative purposes that informed consent usually has, but rather because they are seen by the physician as significant factors in the physician's own decision-making process.

Brody argues that the advantages of this approach are substantial. (1) Rather than informed consent being some sort of alien body patched on to medical practice, Brody asks no more than that "the typical patient-management thought process" be arrayed for the patient, "only do it out loud in language understandable to the patient" (Brody, 1989, p. 8). (2) This approach provides a sense of informed consent that has clear criteria as to what is involved and when the process is adequately completed. (3) It avoids hyperinforming the patient in favor of a structured communication of the basic factors and issues at hand.

Now, as a generic model for the informed consent event, we must reject Brody's strategy, for a variety of reasons. (1) It tends to falsely assume that a physician can legitimately formulate a recommendation for a given patient, in *all* cases, without any prior input from the patient. (2) It ignores the possibility that profound and eminently personal choices may be at hand to which only the patient can speak, and where a recommendation, at any point, would go far beyond the physician's expertise. (3) It would run the real risk of having the physician ignore certain risks or complications that he sees as routine or inconsequential but that might well make the patient pause, or even decide differently. (4) It would tend to diminish the possibility that the patient will rule himself in for hesitancy, ambivalence, or misconceptions. The weight of detail in the first comprehensive disclosure stage is basic to triggering such a rule-in.

However, there seems to be no reason why Brody's model could not incorporate these concerns. In fact, one of the results that we should hope for is that clinicians, as part of their "patient-management thought process," should also be considering the possibility that a recommendation must be preceded by prior discussions with the patient regarding the personal preferences and values that he may or may not have. As a general, preconsent tactic, an enterprise such as getting a "values history" from the patient could be utilized, as some have suggested, although these have been focused on the more specific issues surrounding aggressiveness of treatment.[6] This thought process should also become more patient-centered in the sense of what patients, not physicians, tend to find significant, as well as key to when "similarly situated" patients tend to choose differently, or when "profound and eminently personal" choices are at hand. Thus far, it is not clear that we need disagree with Brody on anything more than emphasis.

The point at which we must disagree with Brody regards whether such a presentation could be sufficient to the other purposes and concerns that we have previously identified. First, though Brody emphasizes that such a process could be documented and be assessed from a legal point of view, as in a suit regarding inadequate disclosure, it surely would not tend to satisfy current legal guidelines, at least in those locales where tort law has been particularly active. We might think of long-shot risks of paralysis or death from a given intervention: the physician may well never have had a patient who experienced these and not find them worthy of either consideration or mention. The physician's patient, on the other hand, might well be given pause when such risks are mentioned and feel unfairly treated or deceived if they are not mentioned and then actually occur. For such reasons we have included our comprehensive disclosure stage to rule out such potential reactions by patients, to give them the chance to throw out the anchor. The physician's legitimate response can still be to try to get the patient to see that the recommended treatment is appropriate even when accompanied by such possibilities, the alternatives being significantly more fraught with peril.

The other reason for not embracing Brody's solution, aside from the fact that it does not satisfy what seem to be current legal requirements in some areas, or satisfy our rule-out agenda, is that it would not provide the patient with the *opportunity* to gain a relatively full understanding of his or her situation and prospects. Although we do not intend to insist on such a result as a necessary condition for an adequate informed consent, we have embraced the view that the opportunity for this sort of result should be provided, either in that the patient actually grasps the content of our first stage or reacts to it by requesting more information and discussion at this level of detail.

For all of this, I believe that Brody's suggestion makes the correct and crucial emphasis in trying to correlate the informed consent event with the actual process of medical decision making. To the extent that we are hoping for effective informed consents, surely the closer the correlation, the more likely they will be provided. Further, as long as we insist that patient-management thought processes be more concerned with and keyed to a patient-centered perspective, with an emphasis on the real choice for the patient, then at least with regard to our second core disclosure stage, the orientation is just right. After all, in a majority of situations, the choice actually presented to the patient is whether to agree to his physician's assessment of his situation and prospects and the response being recommended. In this sense, the core disclosure is appropriately offered in the sense of "this is how I see your situation and the reasons I have for wanting to respond to it in a certain way."

The exact form of a given core disclosure will vary from case to case, and the previous discussion of Brody's recommendation at best gives a generic perspective to guide it. As with our first stage, however, I believe we can identify certain basic guidelines and considerations that should often affect what will actually be said to the patient during this stage.

Considerations in Offering the Core Disclosure

Whereas the first comprehensive disclosure stage emphasized the integrated, detailed provision of information, the core disclosure stage clearly should focus instead on the activity of choice or consent. We might well wish to insist, in fact, on a change in basic terminology—that informed consent be changed to informed choice. I will not make this insistence, simply because the former term has such currency, but the underlying point bears strong emphasis. *Informed consent* seems to embrace the notion that the patient is to be provided with certain information and then is asked to either consent to or refuse what the physician has proposed.

Clearly we should hope for more than this. We should hope not only that the patient will grasp the bits and pieces of information but that he will grasp his condition in an integrated way *and*, to the extent he desires and needs to, reflectively assess such information in terms of his own values, beliefs, and life experiences. Further, to the extent there is a choice between different courses of action, it is the basic lineaments of this choice that we hope patients will perceive, evaluate, and pass on in a reflective fashion. Clearly this could occur, as do most of our decisions in life, on a level of basic information that does not contain anything approaching the level of detail found in the comprehensive disclosure stage. In sum, simply to speak of consent once the information has been provided is to ignore the underlying processes of evaluation, the weighing of pros and cons on a personal level, that we would hope the patient will attempt. It tends to equate information acquisition and the abstract act of consent with decision making, which is simply a delusion. The term "consent" thus tends to ignore that which we might most hope the patients will accomplish, beyond whatever grasp of the bits and pieces they may have gained.

To this end, the core disclosure stage should center around whatever *choice* the patient is being asked to make and the basic reasons the physician has for the choice he is recommending. The choice may involve no more than whether to authorize the intervention that the physician feels is clearly indicated, presented as such by showing the disvalue of not pursuing any treatment and/or the less attractive character of alternative courses of action. To the extent that the physician is himself hesitant, or is aware that similarly situated patients choose differently, then the choice should be arrayed as such, not subsumed under some firm recommendation, even though one might still be legitimately offered. Finally, to the extent that the choice is eminently personal and profound, the physician should emphasize this even if the patient's expectations are not met by such an approach.

Wherever in the spectrum of choice the decision at hand falls, certain emphases and deletions will generally be ingredient in the core disclosure. (1) To the extent a recommendation is being given, this along with whatever sense of a choice is present, should be the focus of this stage, and the physician should straightforwardly proceed to make the case for his preference. We are well past the point for pros and cons merely. (2) Risk disclosure should generally be markedly abbreviated over the previous stage, probably not even mentioning the "minor" risks previously noted. At most, one should mention the overall percentage of occurrence of the group of minor risks and complications, and center on whatever major risks may be present. The physician might well go further and single out only one major risk if that risk is the one the physician is particularly worried about. Also, where the emphasis should fall may well turn on whether a given major risk or complication is reversible or not, with some sense of the percentages and any other accompanying sequelae. It is also appropriate for the physician to perform such abbreviated risk disclosure by reminding the patient of the presumably less attractive risk-benefit profile of the alternatives. (3) As to the contexts of the patient's overall medical condition, and his diagnosis, the potential or actual presence of chronic or terminal illness should also be highlighted and may well become the basic context and coin for expressing the choice at hand, well beyond the immediate therapeutic issue. Many discrete therapeutic situations are part and parcel of a broader, ongoing, and complex course of treatment, and the real decision may be more one of the patient's acceptance of this overall management plan. Individual informed consent events may be useful in reasserting and shoring up the patient's acceptance of and commitment to an overall course of care. In essence, it may well be the latter that the patient is consenting to, or reaffirming his commitment to, and the treatment at hand just part of the package. In sum, it may often be the case that the real choice for the patient is whether to continue with a certain regime of treatment (e.g., intensive care for acute respiratory distress), and the specific treatment being consented to (e.g., insertion of a central line) might legitimately be seen as just part of that overall package, not some new phase of the clinical course. (4) The probable benefits of the proposed treatment should again be qualified, as before, with a sense of any probable limitation to such benefits short of full cure, as should any accompanying major inconvenience that goes along with the treatment, such as a long convalescence, hospital stay, extended rehabilitation, or chronic supportive treatment. Such basic qualifications should not be absent from the core disclosure, as they are essential to the basic meaning and significance of its terms. We must also anticipate that a fair number of patients will attend to and appreciate the content of the comprehensive disclosure only partially. Abbreviation of the core disclosure must be limited by appropriate qualification of the basic information that is still going to be provided. We should, in effect, anticipate that this stage is the one point where the patient will be both attentive and capable of adequately grasping the information provided, and thus retain sufficient detail in response to this.

STAGE III: ASSESSMENT, CLARIFICATION, AND PATIENT CHOICE

The entire informed consent event, thus far, may well occur as a complete monologue, with no input or response from the patient. It might, equally, occur in the form of a single discrete event, with little need for a surrounding process. Given the more modest goals that we have set for the informed consent event, this is acceptable; the primary aims are to give the patient *opportunity* to gain understanding, as well as rule himself in or out regarding other factors such as ambivalence or alarm regarding what he is being told.

At this final stage, however, the patient should be pressed to give some feedback to the physician. This should be done using what Faden and Beauchamp refer to as "feedback testing" or the "feedback loop" (Faden and Beauchamp, 1986, p. 328).

The idea is, in sum, that the patient will, at this juncture, be asked to summarize what he has just been told, and the physician will respond with clarificatory and supplementary remarks. A number of qualifications seem appropriate regarding the character of this stage. (1) At the end of most informed consents, the patient is asked if he has any questions. Anecdotally, it appears that only a few patients respond in detail to this query. It seems worth starting this third stage with such a question, however, as the patient may well be moved to express himself, and the resultant conversation would tend to be just what is hoped for—an interactive communication that proceeds in terms of the hitherto unrevealed perceptions and concerns that the patient actually has. It should be anticipated that the entire third stage may well proceed simply in terms of what the patient says at this point. (2) Whether or not the patient has to be explicitly asked to report back as to what he has just been told, it is helpful and feasible to get the bulk of the core disclosure repeated at this stage, either by the patient or by the physician if the patient responds with less than this. As before, the goal is not necessarily proof of actual understanding, and the patient should be allowed to respond on the level of specificity that he wishes, but this level should be, at a minimum, that of the core disclosure. (3) Letting the patient set the level of detail, the main thrust of the physician's responses should key to this and be especially concerned to clarify apparent misconceptions, or grossly distorted or vague summaries, of the previous communications. The primary aim of this stage is to correct and clarify the patient's actual level of understanding, not necessarily add to it. The physician should not thus simply repeat those aspects of the core disclosure that the patient neglects to mention, but proceed by repeating the patient's account and building upon it. (4) Again it must be emphasized that, in those cases where the physician believes there is a substantial personal choice facing the patient, particularly where either (a) similarly situated patients tend to choose differently, or (b) profound and personal issues are at stake for the patient, the patient should be given some further encouragement to appreciate this choice. As with the prior core disclosure stage, the thrust of this interchange, unless the patient indicates otherwise, should be toward the basic elements of the decision at hand, not on the raw provision or restatement of information.

It should thus be emphasized that this stage is the one place within this event where the patient essentially directs the interchange, in effect dictating the level of detail by his responses, as well as by the sorts of questions he may ask. The physician has already done his duty on an informational level with the preceding two stages, and it is now up to the patient to inject whatever subjective concerns he may have into the event. At some point, we should insist that it is the patient's responsibility to achieve understanding and express personal concerns. The physician should not be forced to play some sort of guessing game or try to force the patient to a level of insight that he may not desire or be capable of. We will discuss the notion of incompetence in the next chapter. The assumption, at this juncture, is that the patient is in fact competent to give informed consent and also competent to reveal the level of detail and insight he desires.

This may well be objectionable to the patient autonomy enthusiasts. I submit, however, that *we should be willing to respect the patient's autonomy also in the sense that he does not want very much detail and is willing to rely on the physician's judgment.* Unless we bias the issue with our own subjective preferences regarding what an autonomous being should do in a given situation, we should be willing to accept even a fairly contentless response and not force the patient to "perform" further.[7]

As a final step, once he has responded to all the patient's statements and concerns, the physician should simply restate his essential therapeutic recommendation and formally solicit the patient's consent to it.

RETROSPECT AND PROSPECT

In this chapter we have attempted to map out a model of informed consent that provides the most effective, efficient, and comprehensive synthesis of our previously noted sources. An event model was chosen as the primary vehicle of informed consent, as opposed to a more conversational or process-oriented model, and the basic considerations and caveats that should guide its provision have been identified and discussed. Though our aims are much more modest than those of certain other commentators, it seems reasonable to believe that the preceding type of event should be markedly more effective in many cases than what is usually offered in practice, and that adequate provision has at least been made toward those goals that we might hope for but rarely seem to capture.

Clearly there is wide variability in the sorts of clinical decisions faced and the patients facing them. Space unfortunately does not allow reference to particular informed consent situations or the charting out and analysis of all the different responses that patients may give to the preceding presentation. There are, however, two further areas of concern that we should specifically reflect upon before completing this discussion: (1) the issue of competence, specifically regarding which patients are to be seen as appropriate recipients of an informed consent; and (2) the issue of exceptions to informed consent, such as emergencies. To the first of these issues, competence to consent, we now turn.

NOTES

1. There will, of course, be instances where multiple diagnoses are at issue, particularly early on in the workup of a patient. Such situations are not rare and will surely complicate the detail of this section. Two caveats seem to bear making. (1) A balance would need to be struck between mentioning all of them, some of which may be theoretical possibilities only, and emphasizing the main possibilities. What would actually be said might be determined by the intervention at issue, especially if it is diagnostic and relates to one of the possibilities. Also, one should be hesitant to assault patients with an extended list of possibilities that will do little more than alarm them and cause needless worry. Our aim throughout is to present important information and encourage patient insight, not to engage in "truth dumping." But (2) it is as potentially disastrous not to identify such uncertainties to the patient up front, as the clinician's credibility, and with it trust, may evaporate if he is forced to modify treatment toward one of the other possibilities later. A good example here would be a patient who presents with shortness of breath and a temperature but also with an X ray containing a suspicious lung opacity. The patient probably has an infiltrate, but this may be superimposed upon a malignancy that also will need to be investigated. To neglect to mention the latter possibility early on will not only strain trust but deprive the patient of time to prepare for the latter discussions. To not even mention the possibility sets the whole process up for failure and may well cause more problems than it solves.

2. See especially the first section of chapter 4.

3. E. Haavi Morreim, personal communication, June 19, 1996.

4. This scenario is discussed extensively in chapter 8 regarding patient waivers of informed consent.

5. This designation is used in passing by Faden and Beauchamp (1986) on page 315. I make no claim as to whether they would tend to accept the "operational" recommendations I am making here.

6. See, for example, Doukas and McCullough, 1991.

7. As long as the situation is one where the clinician sees a certain treatment as "clearly indicated," such latitude should be given to patients. To the extent important compliance issues are involved, or important personal choices are presented, such behavior by patients becomes less acceptable. In this regard, see the discussion of the "waiver exception" in chapter 8, regarding when such behavior by patients should be challenged as unacceptable.

7

The Issue of Competence

The notion of competence becomes a troublesome concept as soon as we recognize that it comes with two quite different meanings, variably emphasized in the literature, and these two conceptualizations pull us in quite different directions.

On the one hand, competence is seen as a *status* concept. Both the law and the new ethos tend to instruct us that it should generally be presumed, and such generally unassessed status confers numerous privileges and rights on patients who are presumed to have it—for example, the right to informed consent and the right to refuse treatment. To presume competence in patients is thus protective of patient freedom and autonomy. This presumption also advances our concern for efficiency because it rejects the need to perform a detailed assessment of the average "alert and oriented" patient as to whether he is capable of performing, or has actually performed, the cognitive and participatory tasks already detailed. Finally, competence in the status sense is clearly an either-or sort of notion. Patients either have such status or they do not.

On the other hand, competence is also seen as an *ability* or *capacity* notion in that a competent patient is deemed to have sufficient ability or capacity to participate in medical decision making. This sense of competence, particularly given the reflections in chapter 3 on diminished competence and the barriers to it, is a spectrum concept. Competent patients fall within a wide range, from the marginally competent to those who are particularly informable, knowledgeable, and reflective about their situation and prospects. A capacity sense of competence thus tends to remain up for grabs however much we are instructed to presume competence in the usual patient, absent significant counterindications. This is so because the patient might still fail to have or exercise sufficient ability in any given instance of information acquisition or decision making.

126

These two senses have led to an extraordinary amount of dispute and confusion in the literature, as well as at the bedside. The presumption of competence runs the risk of false positives. The capacity sense can lead to an overly invasive monitoring and assessment of patient's abilities that have no analogy in the free world and can hardly be attempted even in a small minority of cases. The account offered here avoids opting for one sense of the notion over the other, as previous accounts tend to do. Instead, I propose a notion of competence that incorporates both aspects, status and capacity.

To anticipate briefly, this account proposes to retain the efficient, freedom-protecting presumption of competence that its status sense entails. We will concurrently, however, pursue a quite detailed account of when and how such a presumption may be defeated in favor of a more detailed investigation and assessment of a given patient's actual capacity for and performance of cognitive and decision-making functions. A basic feature of this account will thus regard what sort of clinical factors should trigger a capacity-oriented investigation beyond the usual presumption of competence. Arguably, such an investigation should be conducted when the seemingly alert and oriented patient is refusing an intervention that the clinician sees as clearly indicated for that patient, or when the patient has a history of mental illness. But, given that such factors hardly prove incompetence, we must be as concerned with how to assess such data as with which data legitimately initiate such an inquiry. Past mental illness does not prove present incapacity, nor does disagreement with the clinician as to where one's best interests lie. Our solution will give such factors status only as *triggers*, eliminating them as factors within the competency assessment itself, which they will initiate.

This dichotomy between general status and specific capacity will then resurface within our discussion of the competency assessment itself. That is, once triggered to assess a particular patient's competence, do we assess for some general, across-the-board decision-making capacity, as by some mini-mental status exam, or do we assess in terms of the patient's ability to appreciate the specific decision at hand? Failure at a generic level does not prove the patient might not adequately respond to some specific decision. Equally, generic success guarantees nothing about specific performance. But, alternatively, failure to adequately appreciate and respond to a specific decision-making task does not prove global incompetence. Again, our solution will involve embracing this dichotomy. Within the competency assessment itself, we will advocate using either of these two sorts of tests, depending on the situation and patient at hand. Each one has its place.

As a final anticipation, it should be recognized that an entire book could be written on the notion of competency and how it is to be assessed, informed by the previous source materials. Our account in this chapter can thus not be a complete one. Given our focus on the provision of informed consent to competent patients, we will concentrate mainly on providing a conceptual framework regarding the nature of the presumption of competence and the mechanism by which the clinician may be triggered to go beyond this presumption and actually assess a given patient's competence. As to the specifics of a competency assessment itself, we will provide only a few general conceptual and tactical caveats but not investigate this activity in detail by considering, for example, which mini-mental status exam is most appropriate to use, or how a patient's adequacy at a specific decision-making task is to be evaluated for its success or failure.

To proceed, we must come to terms with the following issues: (1) what a rough conceptual analysis of the concept of competence amounts to, (2) when the presence or absence of competence can generally be assumed without much further investigation, (3) when a patient's competence should be more specifically investigated and evaluated, and (4) what the basic criteria and tactics are for such an evaluation. These goals will be pursued by first referring to what I see as a certain "operational" consensus regarding competence. We will begin by sketching out this consensus and then proceed to modify or augment it as needed, at least in broad outline.

THE STANDARD OF PRACTICE REGARDING COMPETENCE: AN EMERGING CONSENSUS

From ancient times, one basic activity of authors reflecting on morality has been that of "descriptive ethics"—that is, rendering an existing tradition or ethos more explicit. Such descriptive ethics often moves on to "critique" its portrayal, often not in a fundamental sense, where all is up for grabs, but rather in the sense that the concepts and guidelines retailed are given greater precision and sophistication. Such an enterprise is often presented as much more theoretical than it really is, the author not recognizing how indebted he is to prevailing cultural biases and intuitions. Thus Aristotle's *Ethics*, for one example, can be rewardingly interpreted, not as a fundamental a priori ethical system, but as a compellingly insightful description and sophistication of the ethical views of the ancient Greeks.

A similar service has been rendered by a group of scholars regarding our current issue. Loren Roth, Alan Meisel, Charles Lidz, and Paul Appelbaum have worked together over the past couple of decades with particular focus on the notion and practice of informed consent. For our current purposes, one of their articles stands out as just the sort of "descriptive-sophisticative" account that we need. I am speaking specifically of their oft-reprinted 1977 article "Tests for Competency to Consent to Treatment," which does seem to accurately portray and embrace major elements of current practice, along with rendering it more explicit and sophisticated (Roth et al., 1977). In its basic recommendations, it enjoys substantial agreement among commentators on bioethics and thus offers what may be seen as an emerging consensus in this area (Cutter and Shelp, 1991).

This article should not be seen as an exercise in fundamental conceptual analysis. It does not describe and argue for some basic notion of competence and then proceed to identify and discuss the tests for it. Instead, the article basically describes and appears to accept how the issue of competence is usually treated:

> It has been our experience that competency is presumed as long as the patient modulates his or her behavior, talks in a comprehensible way, remembers what he or she is told, dresses and acts so as to appear to be in meaningful communication with the environment, and has not been declared to be legally incompetent. In other words, if patients have their wits about them in a layman's sense it is assumed that they will understand what they are told about treatment, including its risks, benefits, and alternatives. This is the equivalent of saying that the legal presumption is one of competency until found otherwise. The Pandora's box of the question of whether and to what extent the patient is able to understand or has understood what has been disclosed is therefore never opened. (Roth et al., 1977, p. 282)

This seems to be an accurate description of current practice and does, as noted, honor the legal prescription that competence should be presumed unless proven otherwise. In sum, the basic answer to our initial question of what competence is arrives not in the form of a specific conceptual formulation but rather in the sense that competence, whatever it might be, is a thing that is assumed when we are faced with "patients who have their wits about them in a layman's sense." Further, as to when we should be triggered into assessing competence further, two answers are provided. The first answer, *relating to preconsent situations*, is that we do not question competence unless some glaring flaw is noted in the way the patient "modulates his behavior," speaks or reasons, and so forth. As to how this sort of assessment is to be conducted, the article under discussion does not say, but the usual response is some sort of mini-mental status exam that attempts a generic evaluation of the patient's ability to comprehend information and reason, as well as specific questions toward whether the patient is oriented to person, place, time, and so forth.

The basic thrust of the Roth et al. article concerns the patient who has not triggered a preconsent competency assessment, and focuses on the second scenario of when competence becomes an issue during the informed consent process itself. Roth et al. spend the bulk of their article providing a sliding scale of tests for competence, ranging from the simple test of whether the patient can "evince a choice" (i.e., say yes or no to the recommendation offered), to the most elaborate test of whether the patient has a detailed "actual understanding" of the elements of the decision at hand. In between, tests regarding whether the patient's choice was based on "rational reasons" as well as the patient's "ability to understand" are sometimes used, depending on the situation.

Depending on *what* about the situation? Here is the basic contribution of this group, a contribution that fifteen years later seems to enjoy fairly widespread scholarly support as well as to accurately portray how such determinations are dealt with in practice.[1] The crucial move that they make is to contend that the selection of which test to use, from the simple and easily met "evincing a choice" test, to more complex and challenging tests, turns on the degree to which the patient's decision is "favorable" or not. In sum, the more favorable the decision, the lower the hurdle, and conversely.

And how is this "favorability" to be determined? Roth et al., and others, have offered numerous comments and distinctions in this regard, but the most often expressed ground of this determination relates to the risk-benefit ratio of the treatment at issue, what Roth et al. refer to as the "valence" of the decision (Roth et al., 1977, p. 282). Thus to the extent the risk-benefit ratio is favorable, and the patient consents to it, a low threshold test may be used. To the extent such a favorable treatment is rejected by the patient, a relatively more stringent test will be used. Conversely, if the patient refuses an unfavorable or questionable treatment, the test will be low threshold, high if he consents to or demands an unfavorable or questionable treatment (Roth et al., 1977).

And who determines whether a given treatment is favorable or questionable? Roth et al. reply that it is "the person determining competency" (Roth et al., 1977, p. 283), whose identity and training they do not specify. But one assumes they are thinking of either the patient's physician or a psychiatrist consulting to this individual, the psychiatrist basically dependent on the former for the judgment of what treatments are favorable. Favorability, then, is seen as a matter of objective medical judgment.[2]

There is much to recommend this approach. It is surely the efficient way to proceed, assuming competence in most cases where the patient appears basically "alert and oriented" *and*, as is again usually the case, where he accepts his physician's recommendation. This also honors the law's insistence that competence be presumed unless proven otherwise. Further, it is surely an improvement over the older tradition of assuming that patients are generically incompetent to make medical decisions. It also appropriately rejects the traditional notion that the patient is likely to be incompetent if he refuses the physician's recommendations. At least in the latter situation, Roth et al. give the patient the opportunity to prove that his "unfavorable" decision is based on a competent choice, however idiosyncratic, tragic, ill advised, or self-destructive it might appear to the clinician.

Other benefits are claimed for such an approach: the empirical reflections in chapter 3 suggest both the presence of significantly diminished competence in many patients and a lack of comprehensive understanding. Roth et al. point out that this Pandora's box need not be opened in the usual case of the generically alert and oriented patient who accepts recommended treatment. Further, the authors also emphasize the advantage of being able to employ "a low test of competence . . . to find a marginal patient competent so that his or her decision can be honored." Conversely, when a favorable treatment is refused, "even a somewhat knowledgeable patient may be found incompetent so that consent may be sought from a substitute deci7sion maker and treatment administered despite the patient's refusal" (Roth et al., 1977, p. 283).

At some point, however, we must object to all this. The last point particularly, where a "somewhat knowledgeable" patient's unfavorable decision is not honored, seems especially alarming if we value and respect patient autonomy. The whole enterprise starts to look much too expedient. Roth et al. themselves note that "in theory competency is an independent variable that determines whether or not the patient's decision to accept or refuse treatment is to be honored" (Roth et al., 1977, p. 282). But they are surely being accurate as a descriptive matter when they point out that "favorable decisions are more likely to be accepted at face value," whereas "unfavorable" ones are likely to trigger "further investigation" (Roth et al., 1977, p. 282).

Now this focus on "consequences" in competency assessments enjoys a substantial consensus among contemporary writers in bioethics. Perhaps surprisingly, the majority of the authors in a recently published collection regarding competency determinations support this sort of move (Cutter and Shelp, 1991). I say "perhaps surprisingly" as these authors, as well as numerous others, are all devotees of the new ethos of patient autonomy; the list includes such names as Edmund Pellegrino, James Knight, Tom Beauchamp, and John Robertson. And it seems clear that the "appeal to consequences" move fundamentally contrasts with the whole thrust of the new ethos (Wear, 1991). Aside from ignoring the pluralism of values that would undercut the idea that "favorability is an objective medical determination," this whole enterprise could just as easily be seen as only a slight improvement over traditional paternalistic medicine. In effect, the Roth et al. view seems to say, "We will respect your autonomy without question as long as you agree with standard medical judgment, even if you otherwise do not know if you are on foot or horseback. Depart from or disagree with this canon and you will be forced to jump a substantially higher hurdle to retain such respect." It would appear that what we actually have here is the old paternalistic wolf dressed up in sheep's clothing, fangs and claws intact.

COMPETENCE AS BOTH STATUS AND CAPACITY

Another way to put our objection at this juncture is that it seems unjust that patients who decide differently than their physicians will be subjected to a higher level of monitoring of their decision-making abilities than acquiescent patients. Isn't one simply either competent or not? Either a person is sufficiently capable of managing his own affairs or he is not; he is either entitled to the freedom of the community or is not.

It turns out that, even for the law, matters are not this simple. Over the last twenty years, a definite tendency has emerged to move away from a generic, either-or notion of competence to a specific capacity-based notion that focuses on the patient's actual ability to perform the specific decision-making tasks at hand. In nonmedical areas this has led to distinctions where a person of marginal competence may be seen as able to make a simple will but not be allowed to dictate a complex conveyance of property, particularly where substantial assets are involved. One also gets the sense that the same patient might be able to legitimately file for divorce but not be allowed to marry (Wear, 1979). In sum, though the status sense of competence remains in place, its capacity aspect has increasingly risen to the fore, particularly when borderline cases are considered.

In the clinical situation, this tendency arises when the patient's general level of competence and his specific decision-making performance get assessed in diametrically opposite ways. At one extreme, courts have held that even involuntarily committed patients are still at least abstractly entitled to informed consent regarding specific treatments, which they might still be able to legitimately decline. A prime example of this is the involuntarily committed psychiatric patient who refuses neuroleptic medications on the basis that he does not want to be chronically afflicted with tardive dyskinesia. One should be able to imagine such a patient coherently justifying such a refusal in the midst of an otherwise florid psychosis.

At the other extreme, patients who otherwise have the freedom of the community, who might well pass a mini-mental status exam with flying colors, are surely quite capable of incoherently rejecting life-preserving treatment, as when a patient, who makes clear that he does not want to die, rejects the only effective treatment available, whether from fear, denial, or a simple refusal to come to terms with his situation and prospects. One particular patient in my own experience stands out in this regard: a young homeless man with a grossly gangrenous leg, already septic, not only refused amputation but refused to even look at the leg, saying that it would heal just fine if he only washed it more often and got more exercise. In a test of general competence, orientation and alertness, sense of his surroundings, memory, etc. he would have passed with flying colors. He also kept asserting that he would be just fine if only we left him alone, which was definitely false.

Conceptually, there are two basic poles to the tension here—the tension between such "to the task" assessments (capacity) and the generic legal presumption of competence (status). And I submit that much of the confusion in this area comes from different authors emphasizing one pole to the exclusion or at least diminishment of the other.

On the one hand, we have competence as status, the status of being a free person in a free society with the right to conduct and manage one's affairs, with minimal monitoring or impedance. This is the sense of competence that lies behind the legal presumption in its favor and the tendency not to open Pandora's box. Such a status emphasis also is behind the whole thrust of informed consent, particularly in the sense that the patient is the last and ultimate court of appeal concerning what his best interests actually are, any contrary medical judgment in this regard being at best provisional and always defeatable.

On the other hand, there is the growing recognition that many people are not simply competent or incompetent across the board. The floridly psychotic patient may not be disoriented or delusional across the board, and may retain insight and the capacity for judgment in certain specific areas. Alternatively, the generally oriented patient may well fail to accomplish a minimally adequate decision-making process on some specific matter. We have seen that many patients may suffer from diminished competence occasioned by the effects of illness. By definition, all of these individuals are still seen as competent; that is, diminished competence is still competence. But any of them, in any specific instance, might well fail to perform up to a minimally acceptable standard of decision making. This latter sense of competence involves the notion of *capacity* or *ability*, specifically the ability to perform the task presently at hand, to participate knowledgeably in medical decision making. How do we sort these two poles out? A number of options should first be discredited.

(1) We can, at the outset, reject the "sliding scale of competency tests" option,[3] keyed to the favorability of the decision the patient actually makes. The physician may legitimately be triggered into assessing the patient's competency if he feels that the patient's decision is markedly contrary to that patient's best interests. But to make

the nature of that resulting assessment dependent on the physician's own preferences offends against numerous basic principles of the new ethos to which most subscribe—the pluralism of values, the basic value of being treated as competent, as a free agent whose assent must be gained, and the view that competence should be an independent variable, the test of it being the same for all. The use of a notion of competence based on consequences or favorableness thus offends against basic principles and concerns ingredient in the status sense of competence. The reader must understand that I am going against the dominant opinion here, among both clinicians and scholars. As a possible antidote here (if such is needed), I will specifically refer the reader to the work of Allan Buchanan and Daniel Brock (Buchanan and Brock, 1989), which I consider the most forceful and mature presentation of this dominant view.

(2) Another option—and to the extent we are particularly impressed with the specter of "diminished competence" in health care we might well have this tendency—is to test *every* patient as to whether he has attained a sufficient level of "actual understanding" in each instance of decision making. But we have already recognized that people *autonomously* choose to pursue quite varying degrees of understanding, in health care as in all other areas of human endeavor, and that such choices should generally be honored. In addition, there is not sufficient time to conduct such an assessment in all or even a majority of cases. Even if there were, one would expect that patients would resent such a scrutiny, physicians would often not see the point, and, finally, it opens up the Pandora's box that we have numerous reasons to keep closed. Or would we prefer to be running to some surrogate each time a mildly confused, inattentive, or minimally educated patient consents to what the physician clearly feels is medically indicated? Simply as a matter of expediency, the status sense of competence seems clearly preferable, even inescapable, in such instances. Routine assessment of most patients' decision-making abilities is just not an option.

(3) A few thinkers, such as Abernathy, have insisted that competence determinations should be conducted *only* on a generic, global level (Abernathy, 1984). As long as the patient retains sufficient capacity to be entitled to the freedom of the community, his decisions should be respected. This does not prevent the clinician, or family members, from aggressively trying to influence the patient. It insists only that the patient's *ultimate* decision must be honored in the

absence of a generic determination of incompetency. But common clinical experience clearly suggests that generically competent patients may well fail specific decision-making tasks with potentially disastrous results (e.g., the homeless man with the gangrenous leg). Or do we really want to say that the notion of autonomy is so sacrosanct that even questioning it is offensive, and that the physician who feels that the patient is making a tragic, foolish, stupid, or self-destructive decision at most can offer to restate the case, rather than investigate whether there are actual and substantial flaws in the patient's decision-making process itself? To say this would seem to elevate the notion of autonomy to that of a fetish. The notion of competence as capacity cannot be relegated to some subordinate place; clear problems with it can emerge within the context of any informed consent, whatever the generic competency of the patient.

In sum, the notion of competence must be seen clinically as both a status and an ability notion. Its status component is substantial enough to make us insist that it should be an independent variable, at least as far as any appeal to consequences goes, and that any assessment that might result in its loss for a given patient must be as free from subjective bias as possible. Its capacity component, for its part, insists on the equally important fact that the bare exercise of freedom is not all we are worried about here. Part of the value of being free is that we are able to make our own decisions, evaluate information and options as we see fit, and chart our own course. And a basic concern at this juncture is that we know that the capacity to do such things may well be substantially diminished in particular situations, including that of illness.

The basic resolution of the dilemma offered in this section lies in making a sharp distinction between what is allowed to *trigger* a competency assessment—that is, when the presumption of competence is to be overruled—and what is allowed significance within the competency assessment itself. My position will be that the favorability criterion, among others, should be allowed to trigger competency assessments, but it should not be given any significance within the assessment itself, particularly as the determining variable regarding a sliding scale of tests. As in other areas in this book, the aim is to synthesize a compromise of conflicting but legitimate insights and concerns of rival formulations. Regarding such a triggering of the competency assessment, we should first identify the various types of

triggers commonly encountered at the bedside. An unfavorable decision is only one trigger among many.

TRIGGERING THE COMPETENCY ASSESSMENT

To adequately determine whether a given clinical presentation, prior
to or during the process of informed consent, should legitimately trigger a competency assessment,[4] we should first remind ourselves of
what we have already decided to hope for, as well as minimally
require, in the area of patient autonomy and informed consent. On the
one hand, we hope that a patient might actually attain a significant
level of understanding regarding the choices he is facing, evaluated in
light of his own subjective values, beliefs, and life experiences. Toward
this end, we have elected to provide the detailed comprehensive disclosure stage of informed consent, at least toward the possibility that
the patient might rule himself in or out as regards hesitancy, ambivalence, or misconceptions so that further discussion could ensue.
Equally, we have insisted on a core disclosure of the choice at hand so
that the patient might more readily recognize the essential character of
that which he is being asked to authorize. On the other hand, we have
eschewed any requirement for detailed actual understanding, allowing patients autonomously to select the level of understanding and
participation that they prefer. In effect, we have set things up so that
though the minimal "evincing a choice" criterion of Roth et al. will not
be acceptable as satisfying our minimal requirements, a generic rendition of the core disclosure by the patient will often be sufficient, as
long as the patient otherwise modulates his behavior in a normal fashion.

Although we will accept such generic understanding from
patients, we need to set up our model so that we have greater assurance that a given patient actually has the capacity to do what we hope
for. This is *not* to say that the patient actually fulfills our hopes, but at
least that he comes to the informed consent event with the capacity to
do so. It is one thing to accept such minimal behavior from patients as
an autonomous choice that may well not involve much thought, evaluation, or insight. It is quite another to accept such behavior from a
patient who may, perhaps because of the various causes of diminished competence already noted, end up evincing a choice not by
autonomous choice, but because he is, in the present moment, not

capable of autonomous choice. In sum, we need to open up Pandora's box a bit more and somehow gain more surety that the generic assumption of competence is not, in a given case, masking substantial incapacity in the patient.

How might this be *legitimately* and *efficiently* done? To be efficiently done, the assumption of competence must generally hold sway, with further assessment only attempted in a minority of cases. To be legitimate, further assessment must proceed on the same grounds for all patients, free of the subjective biases of others. I suggest that we go back to our rule-out metaphor here. We need to identify legitimate triggers for such a further independent assessment, and these triggers need to be selected on the basis that their presence suggests that the patient may not actually be capable of even pursuing the goods and values for which we have provided the opportunity. That he autonomously chooses not to pursue such goods and values will usually be acceptable; that he is presently unable to do so is not.

What sorts of factors suggest that a given patient may not have such a minimally adequate capacity? Some factors, such as a history of mental illness, dementia, or stroke, are already well recognized as calling for further assessment. Others will become apparent as one goes through the stages of the model just described—for example, when the patient reports ambivalence, hesitation, or alarm. These may well only indicate that the patient needs assistance in evaluating the information and choices presented. But they might also signal the presence of deeper problems that constitute an inability to take advantage of the opportunities being offered. Equally, at the end of the informed consent event, when the patient is asked to report what he understands his situation and options to be, the patient's response may well be so vague, inaccurate, or incoherent that further response is indicated. Again, this might well involve only further clarification and discussion. More fundamental questions about the patient's basic capacities might need to be raised, however. Further, although the informed consent event occurs at one time, observation of the patient by caregivers usually antedates this to some degree, and the ways in which the patient "modulates his behavior," as Roth et al. put it, may well legitimately trigger a further assessment. Finally, any of the factors that potentially cause diminished competence might be present, such as hypoxia, substantial pain medications, inordinate anxiety or fear, and so forth, and further assessment might be indicated by their presence.

Beyond all such examples, the conceptual basis and justification of such triggering need to be clearly and precisely understood. We are attempting to identify clinical factors or realities that *suggest* the possibility that the patient does not have the requisite capacities to pursue the goals of informed consent. This suggestion is then responded to by a competency assessment, and aims at determining, one way or the other, whether the patient does in fact have sufficient capacity. These triggering factors will *not* be part of this assessment itself, given that the patient might still retain sufficient capacity in their presence. They simply raise the issue, dropping out of consideration beyond that. This way of proceeding respects both the status and the capacity senses of competence by not allowing such factors per se to directly discredit a patient's status given that sufficient ability, which the status aspect of competence assumes, may still be extant in their presence. It equally, however, provides us a way to gain greater assurance regarding false positive determinations of competence that a pure status conception of competence tends to allow.

The Favorability Trigger Revisited

And what of the favorability criterion? What role if any should it have, at least at the level of triggering a further assessment? One might wonder how we could entertain allowing it even a triggering function, particularly after what has already been said. In an earlier article, in fact, I myself concluded that such favorability judgments had no place in competency judgments, even for such circumscribed triggering purposes, given that they are in basic conflict with the new ethos, ignore the insight about the pluralism of values, and so forth (Wear, 1991). I now believe such a view to be too purist.

I will first suggest that as long as we do not allow favorability judgments any place within competency assessment itself, then their role is at least rendered much less obnoxious. Also, by recognizing the numerous other triggers noted above, we have returned the focus to that of whether the patient is actually competent to pursue the basic tasks that we have set him. Further, we will thus also test the "marginally competent" patient who makes a *favorable* decision, if he triggers an assessment for some other reason, so we are not biased in favor of the acquiescent patient. Competence thus is returned to its appropriate status as an independent variable.

The reason I think we are obliged to retain the favorability criterion as a trigger rests on our earlier recognition that the clinician often has sufficient grounds to make recommendations concerning the best interests of patients in specific instances. The indicated course of action from a medical perspective is often clear and uncontroversial, need not rest merely on subjective beliefs of caregivers, and usually turns on sophisticated judgments not only about risk-benefit profiles but also on what patients generally want, are able to do and to bear, and what things patients generally find unacceptable or intolerable. However ultimately defeatable by the patient, such conclusions are commonly and legitimately made by clinicians. And the patient who departs from this canon may, in fact, be suffering from factors that undermine the integrity of his or her decision making (e.g., clinically treatable depression) (Jackson and Youngner, 1979). Pandora's box should not be kept so tightly shut that we overlook such common possibilities, and the only indication of them may be in an "unfavorable" response.

It is important to recall that there are certain qualifications regarding the realm in which the clinician can speak with such authority. There are clinical situations where the goods and values at stake are so eminently personal and profound that the clinician cannot legitimately address them without substantial patient input. Similarly, there are clinical situations where similarly situated patients are known to choose quite different options if given the chance to do so. In such instances, there is no favorable choice to appeal to. Favorability, if it is to merit any status at all, must include reference to some reasonable consensus about the needs and typical values of similarly situated patients, and there are times when such a consensus is simply not extant. Finally, Buchanan and Brock appropriately insist that "a patient's rejection of the physician's first choice of treatment should not even trigger an inquiry into the patient's competence," as it may be the case that the patient is still choosing "a treatment that also falls within the range of medically sound options" (Buchanan and Brock, 1986, pp. 85–86).

With these qualifications in mind, the favorability trigger identified by Roth et al. has a legitimate sense and place. It addresses the possibility that a seemingly idiosyncratic, arguably self-destructive choice is not merely different but actually springs from factors that either need to be responded to, such as clinically treatable depression, or may disqualify the patient as a decision maker, at least for the present, such as substantial confusion secondary to his illness. As with the other triggers, however, it would not have any status within the competency assessment itself. Conceptually, the favorability trigger only raises the possibility that the patient may not have sufficient capacity to participate in medical decision making. It must in no way be allowed to bias the decision as to whether or not the patient actually does have such capacity for the simple reason that patients can competently make an unfavorable decision.

Clinical Considerations in Responding to Such Triggers

It should also be stressed that an assessment of competence will often not be the appropriate initial response to any such triggers. Enough has already been said so that the presumption in favor of competence is not seen just as a legal guideline but as a primary clinical desideratum. That is, it is always markedly preferable to have the patient speaking to the issues at hand. Such an event has both intrinsic and consequential value (as chapter 4 detailed). And one way to honor this desideratum is to respond to any such trigger by first attempting to remove or diminish it as much as possible. One might well encounter a trigger that can be sufficiently addressed so the issue does not come to be one of assessing a patient's competency, but at most of assisting a somewhat impaired patient to rise to the occasion.[5] Particularly where matters of profound and personal significance are at hand, the value of such patient participation becomes that much more substantial.

With specific reference to the favorability trigger, the initial response should lie not in a competency assessment but in a blunt statement by the clinician both as to why he is making a particular recommendation and why he sees the patient's response as unfavorable. Further discussion may well result in the trigger's losing its significance, *either* because the patient comes to accept the recommended treatment *or* because the patient proceeds to give a cogent explanation of why he prefers a different course of action. A similar sort of initial corrective response would also be appropriate for the patient who initially gives incoherent or misconceived responses, or appears to be confused or quite anxious. Depression can sometimes be rapidly treated, as can disorienting sequelae such as uremia or hypercalcemia. Equally, obtunding pain medications can sometimes be temporarily reduced with positive results for the patient's degree of alertness. And sometimes just waiting, along with the provision of

care, support, and concern, can remove disabling anxiety, fear, ambivalence, and disorientation. We are thus speaking of *recalcitrant* triggers here, ones that do not respond to attempts to remove or mitigate
them. Such restorative attempts are part and parcel of what it means
to respect and value patient autonomy.

PERFORMING THE COMPETENCY ASSESSMENT

The sorts of triggers just mentioned may become apparent either (1)
prior to approaching the patient for consent—for example, when the
patient appears to have psychiatric illness or seems confused—or (2)
during the process of informed consent itself, as when the patient
makes what the clinician perceives as a markedly unfavorable decision or responds incoherently in the "clarification and assessment"
stage. Recalling the anticipation that our reflections in this area
must remain generic, focusing on conceptual issues and strategies,
not specific tests and tactics, how should an assessment of competency proceed, once triggered?

Having insisted that the notion of competency has both status and
ability (or capacity) aspects, we have two basic choices. One option is
to assess the patient's generic cognitive and decision-making capacities, usually accomplished by some sort of mental status exam. This
option might well lack any specific reference to the decision at hand.
But, as already noted, a person might do well at this level and still fail
miserably in appreciating the specific decision at hand. Conversely, a
patient might do poorly in such an exam but still be able to adequately appreciate and respond to the specific issue. Success or failure
of any such generic competency exam thus leaves open, at least theoretically, the issue of whether the patient can adequately give an
informed consent or refusal to a particular clinical situation.

The other option, of course, is to conduct the assessment directly
in terms of the specific decision at hand, in effect recognizing that
flaws on a generic level might well not be operative in a specific
instance of decision making (e.g., the involuntarily committed psychiatric patient who coherently rejects neuroleptic medications because of
his abhorrence of previously experienced tardive dyskinesia). But the
problem with using the latter sort of test is that we would be testing
for an actual level of performance regarding the decision at hand that
we would not be testing for in a patient who has not otherwise
triggered this assessment. Another patient might be undermined in

his abilities by the very factors with which the present patient has unfortunately presented us. This would seem to be both unfair and misguided.

Again, we arrive at a troubling juncture. If we emphasize generic testing, a patient's flawed response to the task at hand might go unnoted. If we adopt a to-the-task test, we raise the hurdle on a patient who may well be as generally alert and oriented as most other patients who are not tested at all. It would seem that we cannot coherently maintain our dual status and ability notion of competence to the end. We must pick one or the other somehow. Where do we go with all this?

Regarding which of our senses of competence, status or ability, should determine the manner in which such assessments are conducted once triggered, my recommendation is that either may be used, depending on the situation. As anticipated, this account embraces the view that both status and ability are relevant meanings of competence and, given this, both must have a place in triggered assessments of it. I will first address when some sort of generic assessment of competency, like a mental status exam, might be indicated, without or prior to proceeding to a more to-the-task assessment, which would alternatively be conducted in terms of the specific choice at hand.

The Generic Assessment of Competency

As noted, patients usually accept their physician's recommendation, and given the fact that usual clinical practice does not insist on any great deal of interaction from such patients when they do so, I strongly suspect that the majority of patients who trigger a competency assessment will do so outside the bounds of the informed consent event itself. As it should be, such a triggering occurs routinely in an informal way, as caregivers get to know a patient, see how he modulates his behavior, responds to questions asked, and so forth. At such a juncture, given what we have already said, our options for assessment are either to do some generic assessment, such as a mental status exam, or to eschew such general determinations and conduct the assessment whenever a decision is actually at hand via a to-the-task assessment.

The latter option, doing only to-the-task assessments, is too extreme. Whatever the preconsent trigger, minimal investigation may well identify such a degree of disorientation, lethargy, inability to attend to information, both serially and as a whole, or bizarre thoughts about one's situation and prospects, that an attempt at informed consent simply does not make sense. In effect, whatever responses we received from the patient, his ability to pursue the goals of informed consent would simply not be credible. A prime example here would be the somewhat demented patient who can answer individual questions coherently but immediately forgets whatever discussion has gone before. This patient may not even be capable of remembering that he felt alarmed or reticent during the comprehensive disclosure. Nor would he be able to appreciate even a brief core disclosure as one piece. Consent or refusal from such a patient would just not be meaningful. The essay mode of patient understanding and decision making would just not be possible for such a patient.

More generally, one may thus be triggered into assessing competency prior to an informed consent, and there may well be sufficient evidence of disorientation, lethargy, and so forth, that it would make no sense to give the patient the opportunity to attempt an informed consent. Such an attempt would just not be credible. There are, therefore, those patients, such as those whose short-term memory is severely impaired, who are obviously unable to adequately participate in an informed consent once one is triggered to open Pandora's box just a bit. In such instances, a generic evaluation of competence is all that is needed and may be sufficient to defeat the presumption of competence.

Is there any other point at which such a generic assessment is indicated? I can think of one other likely instance—when the patient somehow triggers a to-the-task assessment during the consent process itself and then either fails it or, even if he passes, presents further evidence during the assessment process that he may well be impaired on a generic level. The patient who fails in a specific decision-making task may well be generically impaired in a way that would suggest that further attempts at consent with him are also not appropriate. Such a possibility should be formally addressed as it arises. It must also be recognized, however, that a patient may legitimately retain status as a competent patient but fail to show the requisite ability in some individual situation, as, for example, when diagnosis of a life-threatening malignancy evokes a profoundly recalcitrant denial reaction. Failure of a to-the-task assessment merely raises, but does not at all prove, generic incompetence.

A final note on any such generic testing that does not relate to the actual decision at hand should be inserted here. Such testing is routinely done, usually in terms of some sort of mini-mental status exam. Now there are numerous different psychiatric tests of comprehension, orientation, memory, and so forth. Avoiding a much longer discussion that space restrictions do not allow, I will simply suggest that it is not so much a question of which test one actually employs, or how one proceeds to interview the patient, as it is a question of what one is actually testing for at the generic level. For our purposes, we must keep in mind that we are still testing only as to whether the patient has some minimally adequate *capacity* to appreciate and participate in an informed consent. Though often similar, it is a different matter if one is doing some sort of generic testing to see if the patient should retain the freedom of the community. In the latter sort of investigation, "dangerousness to self or others" often comes in when involuntary commitment or temporary restraint is the issue, and this is not directly relevant to whether the patient can competently approach an informed consent. Equally, flaws of orientation (e.g., as to place and time) may be found but do not have any clear implication as to the abilities at issue. Numerous otherwise "alert and oriented" patients routinely seem to fail to answer such specific questions correctly, and such failures hardly imply that they are incompetent as decision makers. The real issues for a generic assessment of competency are thus not ones of actual factual comprehension or specific orientation, however suggestive such errors may be. Rather, one needs essentially to evaluate "capacities" essential to decision making, such as whether the patient can coherently appreciate and respond to questions and information, whether his memory is essentially unimpaired, whether he is capable of reflecting on abstract matters, and whether he can sustain his attention within a discussion.

To-the-Task Assessments of Competency

Regarding a specific assessment of competency within the frame of the decision at hand, first and foremost it is crucial to emphasize how far the patient will have come at the point such testing will occur. One would be dealing with a situation in which either (1) a patient has modulated his behavior in a sufficiently normal way so that at least informed consent was offered, or (2) some preconsent trigger was identified, but the patient satisfactorily responded to a generic assessment of competency. We would thus say that the presumption of competence has become all the more weighty at the point of a to-the-task assessment, and the burden of proof of incapacity that much harder to satisfy. One way or the other, we will usually be dealing with a patient who is alert and oriented, and is making his wishes known.[6] We will thus have a patient whose status as competent is not just still presumed but has also been given further specific confirmation, and it is the specific exercise of his abilities that is in question. We should first discuss the order of investigation when conducting such a to-the-task assessment since a number of options and considerations present themselves at this juncture.

The Order of Investigation in To-the-Task Testing

The first order of business if an assessment is triggered within the frame of the informed consent itself is, as with a generic assessment of competence, to seek to remove or diminish the factor that is triggering the assessment. In some cases this will already have been attempted (or should have been), as when we are faced with a hypoxic or hypercalcemic patient, or with a patient who is on large doses of pain medication. It should be clear that it will generally be preferable to attempt to remove or diminish such factors beforehand, rather than attempt an informed consent and then seek to respond to such factors only if other triggers appear. In other cases, such triggers (e.g., ambivalence, confusion, incoherent responses, or "unfavorable" decisions by the patient) will appear unexpectedly during the informed consent event itself. Again, the first response to these sorts of triggers should be the attempt to remove or diminish them, either by further clarification and discussion, or by a restatement of the core disclosure.

In the case of unfavorable decisions, a blunt and summary statement by the clinician as to why he finds the patient's decision to be unfavorable, and why another option is seen as markedly preferable from the clinician's point of view, should be offered. Equally, if the clinician sees the patient's view and/or rationale as incoherent, or resting on a false understanding of his situation and prospects, then the clinician should say so, and why, in explicit and blunt terms. Further, a patient who is at risk for having his competency questioned is entitled to know this, as well as know why, specifically, the clinician feels the process is so flawed as to question the patient's status as a decision maker. One may well be concerned as to exactly when and how the patient should be confronted in such a fashion; this will depend on the case and patient at hand. It certainly may not help matters to make the patient defensive by such a confrontation. But neither is it appropriate to dance subtly around the issue and not advise the patient very clearly that serious problems are felt to be at hand.

Such an approach to being triggered by an unfavorable decision by the patient yields a more generic, secondary tactic in approaching to-the-task assessments. Given how far the patient has come, either by not triggering a generic assessment preconsent, or by doing so but passing it, and given that significant effort may already have been made to remove or diminish triggers presented either prior to or during the consent process, the next order of business is to test for whether a flawed consent can be *remediated*. In sum, we should next ascertain whether, by further counseling, discussion, repetition of information, and rationales, we can still assist the patient to accomplish a minimally adequate informed consent. Even if the disconcerting triggers remain intact, can the patient still be assisted to rise to the occasion?

This second suggestion may seem either to go without saying or to avoid the real issue—whether the patient is actually capable of giving an informed consent at this particular juncture. I submit neither is the case. The need for the attempt to enhance or restore autonomous decision making is certainly not the primary instinctive response for many clinicians, particularly those who have little or no faith in it and are presented with a disagreeable, or seemingly incoherent patient. My own experience as an ethics consultant is that I am often called in where there is such disagreement and find that the patient's physician has made little or no attempt to further discuss or investigate the grounds of the patient's recalcitrance, seeming incoherence, or misconceptions. In fact, the physician is often impatient, or even angry, with the patient who is slowing the wheels of progress. So further investigation of the nature and grounds of the patient's problem at least does not go without saying.

Nor is such further investigation an avoidance of the real issue— the patient's capacity to give informed consent. The best and most appropriate test of such capacity is to test whether, with assistance from the physician, the patient's autonomy can be sufficiently restored or enhanced to bring the patient up to the mark. To respond to deficiencies in this regard by simply testing the patient's unassisted level of understanding, insight, clarity and coherence of rationale, etc. is, to my mind, just another instance of inadequate respect for the person's autonomy, his *status* as an otherwise free agent, as a person with his own unique values, beliefs, and life experiences. At this point in this work, it should be clear that intense and, at times, extended proactivity is the required response of the clinician. Whether the assessment has been triggered by a history of mental illness, or present confusion, or an unfavorable response, deficiencies in decision making by a patient are often eminently remediable. Further, given the intrinsic value and status of autonomous patient decision making, such proactive and enhancing efforts should always be the primary response—the basic test—at such a juncture. And more basically: such proactivity may well be the most important and core sense of why a process of education and counseling should surround the informed consent events that we are mainly putting our money on.

Another conclusion drawn from my experience as an ethics consultant is also relevant. Most cases that I am called to consult on involve disagreements among staff and either patients or families as to how to proceed. Now, as an academically trained philosopher, my early bias was that such disputes would usually turn basically on differences of personal values and beliefs, which must somehow be negotiated out, or at least clarified. At that time, I thought that the facts of the matter would be less pivotal, facts being, for most academic philosophers at least, rather plastic as to the interpretation of their significance and value. They are thus much less likely to be the needed focus in gaining a resolution to disagreements, the appropriate response instead being some sort of values clarification.

The true ground of most such disagreements turns out to be otherwise. The majority of them dissolve once the parties concerned have taken the time to rediscuss and clarify the facts of the matter. Once these are agreed on, which usually occurs with further effort, agreement as to how to proceed generally occurs naturally and quickly. The sources of such factual misunderstandings are mainly twofold: (1) an inadequate or flawed presentation by the clinician to the patient or family—a presentation that is too vague or technical and/or lacking an attempt to assess what the patient or family actually heard as a result; or (2) an idiosyncratic, subjective misunderstanding by the patient or family of the situation, options, and prospects at hand.

Regarding the first source, these experiences have had a strong effect on the design of the informed consent event previously offered, the uniform need for which may be received in terms of the principle of doing it right the first time. As to patient and family misunderstandings, my experience is that even when the clinician does do it right the first time, their understanding of the situation often relates predominantly to prior, often disanalogous experiences that they or their loved ones have faced and only secondarily to what they have been told by the clinician. Particularly when these past experiences, such as the death of a loved one, have been especially profound, the task of the clinician in generating true insight may be formidable and still fail even if quite competently and diligently pursued. In my experience the typical case arises when a patient is deathly ill and he or the family has the prior experience of a loved one who was treated aggressively, died anyway, and in addition underwent a much more prolonged, pain-filled dying process. It often takes a great deal of discussion to get such a patient or family to accurately see that the present situation is markedly disanalogous, if such is the case. And the danger *here* is that a superficial subservience to patient or family autonomy becomes operative by accepting directives based on such misconceptions or fears. An intense, at times quite extended, attempt to clarify and communicate the facts of the matter is the needed response.

So in approaching to-the-task assessments of competency one first seeks to remove or diminish the triggering phenomenon, and second one attempts to restore or enhance the patient's autonomy. There is certainly no formula as to how such a process should be conducted at the bedside, but clarification of both the facts and rationales, drawing the patient out as to what he perceives to be the problem, his feelings and concerns, is surely a basic part of it. Hopefully, however disconcerting the initial triggers, a successful conclusion will result.

Negative Findings in To-the-Task Assessments of Competency

Prior to any attempt at informed consent, a patient may be found to be so incapacitated that no such attempt should be made, as when unconsciousness or gross confusion is present. Such a state of affairs may also arise within the consent process, as when a patient triggers further assessment and similar high degrees of confusion or abnormal ideation are encountered and turn out to be intractable. The further suggestion is that the clinician then attempts to assist the patient to rise to the occasion. But what if such corrective efforts do not succeed? At what point, regarding a to-the-task assessment, can one legitimately conclude that the patient has failed the task and refer matters to a surrogate decision maker?

Patient Performance within a To-the-Task Assessment

The basic ground for a negative finding in to-the-task assessments relates to the *process* characteristics of the patient's response to the decision-making task at hand. Specifically, if the patient's response, beyond all efforts at remediation, remains essentially confused, or incoherent, then incompetence—specific incapacity to the task at hand—may be concluded. The patient who is refusing the only life-saving therapy available but is still maintaining that he wants to live is a pertinent example. Equally, the patient who repeatedly refuses and then accepts care, or continues to give ambivalent responses, may well be legitimately determined to be incapacitated on the level of a to-the-task assessment.

Glaring failure in this process sense of performing specific decision-making tasks may not be present, however, but disconcerting failures to perform in another sense may be—namely, the patient may retain a substantially false or misconceived sense of his situation and prospects. A common source of such a result is denial.

Now, as we are embracing a "capacity to the specific task at hand" criterion for such competency judgments at this juncture and have also embraced the idea that patients can autonomously choose to participate only minimally in decision making, it would seem that the assessment at this point should not be performance based in the sense of the patient's actual grasp of information. It would be unfair to numerous patients to hold them to a higher level of actual understanding than we will insist upon with the patient who does not trigger such an assessment. The patient with a history of mental illness, for example, should not be forced to jump a much higher hurdle than a patient without one.

It would seem difficult, however, to separate out factual appreciation at this stage, as we would be conducting the assessment in terms of the actual details of the decision at hand, not the more generic sort of competency assessment, such as by mental status exams. One would, of course, focus more specifically on the essential details of the patient's situation and prospects—that is, the detail provided in the core disclosure. Given all that has gone before, the detailed, serial understanding of risks, benefits, and options that empirical studies of informed consent usually focus on should not be the focus of testing. We have already accepted the idea that many competent patients will perform only moderately well at best at regurgitating such a list. At most we should insist on the level of detail of the core disclosure.

Such a further performance-based test would seem inescapable. At some point the real apparent flaw in decision making on the patient's part may well be essentially factual, not one of coherence of rationale (as when a patient both indicates he wants to live and rejects the only effective means to accomplish this). Either from denial or some other factor, a patient might simply be deciding on the basis of a patently false understanding of the facts at hand, as in my earlier example of the man who rejected amputation for a gangrenous leg, falsely asserting that more baths and some exercise would cure the condition.

I thus submit that aside from dramatically confused, ambivalent, or incoherent responses by the patient, a false understanding of the facts at hand must also be allowed to justify a negative finding regarding competence in a specific patient. This is the last possibility envisioned in the order of response in to-the-task testing and can be legitimately contemplated only with a number of caveats.

(1) Indicting a patient's competence on the basis of false understanding raises the hurdle higher than that which most patients are expected to attain. This is unavoidable but must be minimally done, keeping at most to the essential facts of the decision at hand as detailed in the core disclosure. To ask for more detail than this would routinely disenfranchise patients for not performing on a level of understanding that we have good reason to believe many nontriggering patients do not attain. That we may and should insist on even a core disclosure level of detail is justified by the insight that failure at such a basic level of understanding may well occur, become apparent, not be remediable with further discussion and clarification, and be the ground of incoherent or unfavorable decisions by the patient. That we have insisted that an extended, proactive attempt by the clinician should ensue in response to such a presentation makes its incorporation less egregious.[7]

(2) Reflection on the nature and significance of denial within competency assessments is needed.[8] On the one hand, denial in the face of disastrous news or situations is perfectly normal and, though there can come a point at which it becomes pathological, that claim will often not be sustainable, at least in the sorts of situations envisioned. Nor need it be; we do not need to find such denial pathological to hold that the false understanding of the facts that it generates and supports may render the patient's decision making intolerably flawed. A false understanding of the essential facts is simply that, and renders the incorporating decision making process invalid.

(3) To rest an incompetency judgment on such a false understanding of the facts should also be pursued cautiously in another sense. The level of detail in to-the-task assessments, as noted, should go no further than the level of the core disclosure. A further appropriate guideline should be that the facts falsely understood should be so pivotal to the decision at hand, and so directly causative of the triggering incoherence or unfavorable quality of the decision, that the decision making is impeached as a direct result. It should not be enough to show the patient has misconceptions. Such misconceptions must be shown to be markedly recalcitrant to further discussion and counseling *and* central to the decision at hand.

(4) Incompetency judgments at this level, even if all the preceding attempts at clarification, counseling, and remediation have failed, should not necessarily issue in immediate treatment over the patient's objections. One must also be able to justify such an extreme response on the basis of substantial risks of mortality and morbidity for the patient if one does not act. If, in other words, the intervention can be put on hold without major negative effects to the patient, then it should be withheld as time and further discussion may yet resolve the problem. Some patients just need time to sit and stew.

(5) It should finally be the case that if the patient has come so far as to be judged otherwise alert and oriented, having either passed a generic assessment or not having triggered one, has withstood all attempts to remove the triggering phenomenon and restore or enhance autonomy, and has not clearly been found to be incoherently making the decision, then barring a true emergency, provision of therapy over the patient's protests should probably only occur on the basis of further review by an independent body. Such a required concurrent review might be accomplished by another attending physician or one's chief of service, or an ethics consultant or committee, if not a court of law. The scenario envisioned here is simply too profound and disconcerting, particularly in a free society, to allow any one clinician to unilaterally exercise such an option without confirmatory independent review.

SUMMARY REMARKS

The issue of patient competence is thus radically affected by the value that we, as free men and women, place on the notion of patient autonomy. In the vast majority of clinical interactions with patients, clinicians should thus assume its presence and honor the patient's wishes, without further investigation of the level of understanding and reflection that may be involved. Beyond this, there are clearly many instances where a patient is not competent to participate in decision making in any meaningful sense, and judgments to this effect can often be legitimately made by a physician at the bedside.

In only a small minority of situations, then, does patient competence need to become a real issue. We have attempted to sort out some rough guidelines regarding appropriate clinician behavior at such junctures. Again, given the value of patient autonomy, insight into the pluralism of values, and so forth, we have concluded that attempts to remove triggering phenomena, along with attempts to restore or enhance autonomy, are initially requisite, at times meriting extraordinary efforts by the clinician. We have also sought to distinguish all such triggers as only calling for such an assessment, not as having determinate status within the assessment itself. As to such assessments, once triggered, they may well be conducted on a generic level, as with a mental status exam, or on a specific to-the-task level, internal to and in terms of the actual decision at hand. On both levels of assessment, the main focus of concern would regard the character of the patient's decision-making process and ultimately rest on process sorts of considerations, i.e. the consistency and coherence of the patient's decision making, not simply factual recall or insight. This may be found to be flawed generically, as when the patient is irremediably confused or incoherent, or specifically, as when the specific decision making is flawed, as in an incoherent response. Only at the very end of such evaluations and responses did we envision that intractable false beliefs about basic matters might also justify a verdict of incompetence, and that verdict was seen as often requiring independent review.

To move on, there are other instances in which an informed consent may well not be offered to patients—for example, in emergencies or when the patient explicitly waives the right to informed consent. We must now seek clarity in these situations as well.

NOTES

1. See especially Cutter and Shelp, 1991.
2. One might read these authors as saying no more than that for a patient's decision to be "favorable" it must agree with the clinician's specific

preference. Although they are not clear on this, I do not believe they intended something so minimal and subjective. Objective medical judgment avoids this, as it can and should recognize that similarly situated patients can reasonably have different preferences among legitimate modalities, whatever the clinician's specific preference might be.

   3. Allen Buchanan and Dan Brock have offered a more recent account of competence that retains the "sliding scale of competency" test, keyed to the notion of "favorability," as do Roth et al. Though I reject this option for the aforementioned reasons, insisting that favorability can be only a *trigger* for competency assessments, their account provides a much more detailed argument for this sort of view, and the reader is strongly encouraged to refer to their work *Deciding for Others*, especially their first chapter, for a forceful, alternative treatment of these issues (1989, pp. 17–86). See also my further argument regarding "favorability" in this chapter.

   4. I had once believed that this notion of triggers was original on my part. I have subsequently found other authors who have independently suggested it. See, for example, Haavi Morreim's discussion of "suspicion-triggers" (Morreim, 1991, pp. 121–22, note 4). See also Jonathan Moreno's use of this strategy with adolescents (Moreno, 1989). It is also a major feature in the first chapter dealing with competency in Brock and Buchanan's *Deciding for Others* (1986, pp. 17–86).

   5. It may be objected that such a response can take time and may run the risk of heightening the patient's morbidity and mortality. However, even increased morbidity and mortality do not necessarily rule out such an attempt. Given our recognition that patient participation in decision making itself has both intrinsic and instrumental value, the disvalue of risking morbidity and mortality to the patient by waiting for sufficient decision-making capacity may well be seen as acceptable, all things considered. This would depend on how significant the threat is to the patient and how important such participation is in a given case.

   6. Such an alert and oriented patient may not always be making his wishes known; he may well be so ambivalent or hesitant as to be unable to evince a choice. This should generally be responded to by further clarification and assessment; it may also result in the patient's electing to waive the right to a full informed consent, trusting instead in the clinician's or a surrogate's judgment, an exception to informed consent that is discussed in the next chapter.

   7. The argument here, or lack of it, may well strike some readers as philosophically insufficient at best. It is still the case that we would be requiring a level of factual understanding at such a juncture that is not required of nontriggering patients, and we have good reason to suspect that most patients will have some flaws in understanding, certainly in grasping all the detail, sometimes on a more basic level. In a more extensive deliberation, I would

attempt to offer a Rawlsian sort of argument in favor of the point that a neutral, rational observer would tend to accept the notion that triggering individuals are legitimately asked to perform at a heightened level to protect against the possibility that factual misunderstanding may well be the root cause of the triggering presentation and constitute what amounts to an essentially inadequate decision-making process. I am not sure that this argument would tend to be supported by all, particularly advocates for those with a history of mental illness, who would be routinely triggering to-the-task assessments. Perhaps some triggers, such as a history of mental illness, should be allowed to trigger only generic assessments, not to-the-task ones. But the options and considerations here are just too byzantine to sort out in the space available to us.

    8. See Roth et al. (1982) for an extensive discussion of the issue of denial in competency judgments.

8

Exceptions to Informed Consent

Following legal developments in the United States, there are certain well-recognized types of situations where informed consent need not be solicited from the patient. The exception based on the incompetence of the patient has already been discussed in the previous chapter. Aside from patient incompetence, there are three other legally sanctioned types of exceptions: (1) in an emergency, when there is insufficient time to pursue an informed consent, at least if one is to avoid significant morbidity and mortality to the patient in the interim; (2) when a competent patient waives the right to an informed consent and consents to what the physician wants to do without further information; and (3) when the physician claims the therapeutic privilege not to inform the patient on the ground that the informing process itself would likely harm the patient in an unacceptable way. We will deal with each of these possible exceptions in this chapter, being particularly concerned to state their sense and justifying conditions as specifically as possible, lest such exceptions come to undermine the rule of gaining informed consent.

THE EMERGENCY EXCEPTION

In general, the emergency exception may be stated as follows: "If informed consent is suspended in an emergency, it should be because the time it would take to make disclosure and obtain patients' decisions would work to the disadvantage of some compelling interest of patients" (Appelbaum, 1987, p. 68). Specifically, an emergency situation that would legitimately justify withholding the attempt to gain an informed consent would involve the following factors: (1) there must be a clear, immediate, and serious threat to life and limb; (2) the

156

treatment that will be provided without informed consent should be the one that most practitioners would tend to recommend for the condition, i.e. one that is in keeping with the standard of practice; and (3) the time it would take to offer an informed consent would significantly increase the patient's risk of mortality and morbidity, either because these are presently occurring or because the effectiveness of a given treatment will be significantly diminished if not immediately instituted.

Now, the appropriateness of withholding informed consent will lessen as the situation recedes from the above characterization—for example, to the extent the threat is not so clear, immediate, or serious. And, as usual, we should not expect much more specific operational guidance from the law in such unclear situations. But the way in which the emergency exception is usually treated in the law seems to make it mainly a question of medical judgment that will seldom be in danger of legal censure after the fact. The legal account of the grounds for this exception keys to the notion of *presumed consent*—namely, that it is a safe assumption that patients would want whatever is "medically indicated" to minimize or prevent injury, stop the progression of disease, sustain life, relieve pain and suffering, and so forth. Once the notion of presumed consent is accepted, then the rest of the issue becomes one of medical judgment by the clinician on the spot, based on three related judgments: (1) that a specific form of therapeutic response is medically indicated; (2) that the effectiveness of this response will be significantly compromised to the extent that time is taken for informed consent or the assessment of patient competence; and (3) that additional morbidity and mortality are likely to affect the patient to the extent one pauses for informed consent.

It would thus seem to be the case that if the emergency response provided satisfies the usual standard of practice guidelines, and delay can legitimately be seen as potentially compromising its effectiveness, then a physician can comfortably proceed to invoke the emergency exception with no attempt to inform or gain consent from the patient. There appear to be no cases where suit or sanction has been brought against a physician if these conditions are present to some significant degree. As a legal matter, then, the emergency exception would seem to be unproblematic in most cases.

But are there *ethical* issues of concern here, even if legally the physician may be comfortable in invoking the emergency exception as he sees fit? Four major ones merit review.

The Competing Value of Informed Consent

As informed consent is itself a "compelling interest" of patients, the interests appealed to by the emergency exception may not be as compelling as it is, and thus the appropriateness of delaying treatment for "further discussion" should be contemplated as potentially appropriate even in an emergency. Such an interest in informed consent would itself be particularly compelling if some especially "personal and profound" choice were at hand. In this regard, a threat or risk to a compelling interest of a patient can come in the form of straightforward morbidity and mortality, options and opportunities compromised or lost, or simply that the patient is deteriorating in the interim; but such interests vary markedly as to how clear, immediate, and serious they are; equally, the potential effectiveness or risk of the treatment to be imposed will vary.

That such variables exist and might well affect the legitimacy of a given emergency exception is clear in the abstract; what is not clear is whether and how this insight can be clinically operationalized. There is always the danger that a given clinician will insufficiently value informed consent, or not appreciate the "value-charged" character of what he wants to do, and invoke the emergency exception where this is questionable. I submit, however, that it will not do to dig further and somehow complicate the reflection and justification necessary to choose the emergency exception; we should avoid hamstringing the clinician in ways that would only increase morbidity and mortality. This is so particularly because one seldom hears of any retrospective complaint about its usage. This seems to be the case as the initial response in emergencies often is essentially twofold: (1) to treat obvious problems (e.g., diminish unstable angina) and (2) to stabilize the patient for further workup on the floor or in the intensive care unit (e.g., assess cardiac function with an angiogram). More profound interventions, such as major surgery, are seldom elected as part of the emergency unless the indications are clear, as, for example, where gross internal bleeding demands immediate surgical exploration and response. In effect, wide latitude in treatment response in emergencies is itself limited by the initial need to stabilize and further work up the patient. One might, in sum, produce a long treatise on the potential ethical problems submerged by appeal to the emergency exception, but until such problems become frequently emphasized retrospectively by patients, it seems prudent to leave them submerged.

The ethical point is that the presence of sufficient legal justification for the emergency exception does not necessarily mean that the emergency exception should be invoked. The presence of profound and personal choices might still call for an attempt to address them, with immediate treatment held in abeyance.

The Time Factor and Treatment Refusals in an Emergency

A second issue in any acute situation concerns whether the patient is competent to receive disclosure and make decisions. The time problem emerges because a patient's compelling interests might be jeopardized if we pause to assess competency. This issue gets particularly poignant when a patient presents with a life-threatening condition to an emergency room and is rejecting treatment in some way.

Again, I submit that this raises issues that are hard to operationalize in the emergency situation. Not only would an attempt to assess competence expend precious time to the patient's harm, but attempting to respond to such refusals, which may amount to no more than a confused, agitated patient fighting back against the unknown, would be either hopelessly brief or carry their own jeopardy. As was noted in the previous chapter, some patients may be clearly confused or obtunded; some, on the other hand, may appear rational and calm, and the latter generally tend to give clinicians pause in an emergency when they refuse care. The borderline case where competence is not clear and the threat is immediate and serious, however, would seem appropriately treated under the emergency exception, the appeal being to presumed consent and its underlying justification, that people usually want treatable illness treated, pain and suffering relieved, and so forth. Here, as in many other areas, I believe we must accept Franz Ingelfinger's suggestion that the only real protection is the conscientious and compassionate physician, and reflection on the merits of such cases best occurs after the fact.

The Abbreviated-Consent Option

The use of an abbreviated informed consent, including the solicitation, has been suggested as an option in some instances (Appelbaum, 1987, p. 69), including the solicitation of a bare consent to treat without further explanation. I believe there are a number of problems with any such suggestion. First, the status of any such gesture will immediately become problematic if the patient in some way refuses to give such a generic consent. Does one then hold treatment and pause for the sort of competency assessment, as well as further discussion and counseling, discussed in the previous chapter? This seems sensible only if the emergency is significantly short of the usual clear, immediate, and serious threat variety. One should not exercise this option unless one is legitimately prepared to engage in the further assessment and discussion that would usually accompany it, particularly if a refusal emerges. In sum, one should not make such a gesture unless one is prepared to follow through on it.

A second problem with abbreviated consents in emergencies is that the solicitation of a bare informed consent seems meaningless in such a situation. It rests on no information about the choices at hand and assumes some degree of competence in a situation where not only are the patient's abilities in this regard quite unknown, but there may well be substantial prima facie grounds for doubting them, such as shock, hypoxia, or blood loss.

One might respond that the attempt to gain an abbreviated informed consent, perhaps by provision of some sort of core disclosure, may make sense. But again, if the threat is clear, immediate, and serious, and the intervention clearly indicated, this would seem inappropriate, at least in the sense that one is seeking *consent*, because one may be loath to have further discussion and counseling, or attempt to assess competence, if the patient somehow balks at consent. In sum, if one cannot adequately follow through with the consent process if a problem emerges, one should not start it. If time is available for it (i.e., serious morbidity and mortality are not threatened by taking the time), a version of the core disclosure that advises the patient as to what is going on and what will be done about it may well be appropriate, but this should be offered not as a solicitation of consent but rather as telling the patient what is happening and what will be done about it. In sum, we might well provide the patient with an abbreviated disclosure, but not ask for consent.

Emergency Response in the Context of Terminal or Severe Chronic Illness

A final point regarding consent in emergency situations concerns the use of aggressive therapy in patients with *known* terminal or severely debilitating disease. Patients are often aggressively treated in emergency situations when everyone on the spot has severe doubts as to whether the patient would want such management. The patients at issue here include the terminally ill, such as a patient with metastatic disease who presents in any of the many ways that such people tend to die, or the severely debilitated patient, such as one with severe chronic obstructive pulmonary disease with an acute infiltrate. And the "choices" in such an emergency are all quite problematic: one can opt to stabilize the patient, which may lead to a dying patient who is bound to a ventilator for the duration, or one can withhold therapy on a patient who might have some chance of gaining some remaining "good time" if aggressively treated. I submit, however, that to attempt to have the discussion that is needed with such a patient at such a time is not a meaningful option. Perhaps one of the most farcical things one can witness in a modern hospital is the attempt by a physician to ask such a patient, often in pain, confused, and with metabolic anomalies, if he wants his "heart restarted if it stops" or wants us to "beat on your chest if you die."

But the basic point in such instances is not whether and how the emergency exception should be employed. Such clearly anticipatable end-stage scenarios should be identified and discussed with such patients prior to their occurrence. Preventive ethics is thus the appropriate response (Wear, 1989). One should not shrink from discussing distressing matters out of some superficial compassion for the patient and end up brutalizing him in ways that most people would not want. The best way to deal with ethical issues is often to see them coming and prevent their occurrence.

In the absence of such preventive measures, reliance on the emergency exception's option of aggressive treatment seems appropriate. A quick or abbreviated attempt to ascertain the patient's wishes while he is in extremis will generally not bear analysis, as an act either of consent or of compassion. Stabilization of the patient, with full treatment to the point of intubation in an intensive care unit, should generally be pursued. The trick will be to ensure that one has the option of discontinuing life support if the patient's prognosis turns out to be as bleak as was initially feared, or clear prior statements against such maintenance turn out to be extant. The aggressive posture here includes the injunction not only to treat aggressively when in doubt but also to discontinue aggressive therapy when such treatment is retrospectively determined to be contrary to the patient's interests or clear wishes. One stance implies the other.

The essential point of our discussion of the emergency exception is thus that it can almost always be legitimately and comfortably invoked as a legal matter on objective medical grounds. Allied to this, the further suggestion is that abbreviated gestures at informed consent, or concern about abuse in rare cases, should not be allowed to dampen the clinician's tendency to exercise this exception when medical judgment indicates. The stakes can be too high to muddy the waters in such cases, and consents gained without knowledge, or attempted in situations where the lack of a resulting consent should not be allowed to delay treatment, should not be attempted. As to those paradigm instances where aggressive treatment appears questionable at best, they should be addressed beforehand, when the patient has his faculties and has the time to be adequately informed and think through the options involved.

THE WAIVER EXCEPTION

The least troublesome and most straightforward of our three exceptions would appear to occur when a clearly competent patient elects to waive his right to an informed consent and simply consents to whatever the physician believes is indicated. This exception is the least troublesome because such a waiver can be seen simply as an autonomous act by the patient, as legitimate as any other decision. It would also not seem that troublesome given our strong suspicion that many patients exercise this option sub rosa—by not really attending to the details of the informed consent, waiting for the punch line, and accepting whatever the physician recommends. To the extent we are troubled by explicit waivers, we should be as troubled by the much more common inattentive patient.

The law, at least, seems to have few problems with such patient waivers per se and seeks only to ensure the integrity of the process. Faden and Beauchamp emphasize that a person can "effectively waive a legal right only if the waiver is informed, reasoned, and voluntary" (Faden and Beauchamp, 1986, p. 38). These conditions would appear to be met when the patient who seeks to waive informed consent is aware that he is giving up something that he has a right to, has some reason for waiving the right, and is not being pressured or intimidated by anyone to do so. As a practical matter, at least on the score of being legally legitimate, the preceding entails the following: (1) the patient must be counseled that he has a legal right to informed consent; (2) his reason(s) for not wanting informed consent should be documented; (3) the physician should probably not be the initiator of the discussion about such a waiver lest some party (including the patient) later questions whether there was something inappropriate about it, or claim it was gained via some sort of subtle intimidation or manipulation; and (4) the generic competence of the patient should be attested to.

As with the emergency exception, we may, however, have serious ethical difficulties with the waiver exception even if its legal status is generally unproblematic. The source of such a waiver can, of course, be quite rational—for example, when the patient simply feels unable to appreciate and pass on the complexities at hand and is quite willing to trust in the physician's judgment. This is also the case when a patient suspects bad news and feels unable to deal with it at the present time. Not only are such feelings rational, but waivers generated on the basis of them are as autonomous as any other acts.

I would submit, however, that such waivers should generally be received in a skeptical fashion on a clinical/ethical level, however rational and voluntary they may appear to be. Surely we have come too far not to be concerned about a patient's refusing such an important task as participating in decision making. Too many goods and values may be at stake to accept such a decision lightly. It is worth emphasizing that however much we may respect autonomy, that does not mean we would not want to counsel the patient against what we see as an unwise choice. And, given all that has gone before, it is fair game to hold that refusing to participate in informed consent is itself, prima facie, an unwise choice. Further, there are clearly cases, such as the following, where such a waiver would appear to be quite unwise or inappropriate.

(1) An obviously terrified patient may use the waiver to escape hearing about what he fears. Aside from the fact that such fear merits clinical response (part of which would involve discussing what he fears and whether such fears are accurate), the patient may also be burdened by wholly inaccurate fears, thinking his situation is much worse than it actually is. One might conversely be dealing with a patient who is proceeding with an overly cavalier or optimistic sense of his situation and prospects and needs to be similarly disabused of this.

(2) The patient may well be in one of those situations where eminently "personal and profound" choices are at hand, or where "similarly situated patients" choose differently. To force the clinician to make decisions as though there were some objective standard to appeal to, or as if the physician were adequately aware of the

patient's values and beliefs to make such a profound and personal choice for the patient, is to perpetuate a delusion; it should thus be resisted.

(3) There is an element of refusing to take responsibility for one's life involved in such a waiver that is objectionable on a number of scores. It may signal a patient who will be quite passive regarding treatment, and this itself may be detrimental to its efficacy, as when compliance and self-monitoring are important. Equally, it may signal a patient who falsely believes that medical decisions are matters for experts, generated solely on objective grounds and without any need for correlation with the patient's values and beliefs (here, even if the decision at hand is quite straightforward, objection to a waiver from the clinician might be appropriate since such a tendency might be detrimental in a later situation). Further, there may be an attempt to place all the responsibility on the physician, and the physician might legitimately (and prudently) refuse to accept this. The physician who accepts a Godlike status from such a patient is being set up for a fall, perhaps even a legal suit, when it turns out that he did not have the requisite divine capacities, e.g., omniscience or omnipotence.

(4) There are surely situations where the attempt at waiver flows from an arguably "pathological" state that itself merits clinical response. I am thinking of the terminally ill patient who is so completely stuck in denial that he cannot bear to hear anything about what is happening to him and may be doing everything he can to ignore or downplay it. For us to accept that such denial responses are natural occurrences within a patient's evolving response to the threat of serious or terminal illness hardly also entails that we are obliged to accept such reactions to the bitter end, particularly when they are having serious negative repercussions on the lives and fortunes of the patient and/or his loved ones. Not that we will necessarily grab such a patient and do what we think best to him. But we might well decline to accept a waiver that seems to flow from such a source and attempt to get the patient to consider his situation and prospects specifically.

For all of the preceding, however, I would stop short of concluding that waivers are a bad idea in most instances and should usually be opposed by the clinician. As mentioned, our strong suspicion is that many patients exercise a *sub rosa* form of waiver by not listening to informed consents and waiting for the punch line, which they tend to accept uncritically. Given this, we should either (a) be challenging them also when we suspect such behind-the-scenes behavior, or (b) should accept a patient's waiver when he is candid and insightful enough to offer one. The former reaction would not seem feasible given the number of patients who appear not to be listening. So it would seem that we should honor most waivers rather than inflict extra scrutiny on patients who are just being more candid than most.

We can do better than this. In general, I would suggest that any attempt at waiver by a patient, explicit or sub rosa, should minimally involve some exploration of why the patient wants to do this. Some responses might be accepted at face value without further comment or investigation, as when a patient wants to defer to the physician's judgment and the situation is one where the treatment is clearly indicated and does not involve either basic choices for the patient or threats to well-being that the patient should know about up front. Equally, the patient who indicates that he is presently unprepared to deal with the gory details might be *temporarily* accommodated in this, as long as, again, immediate therapeutic response is clearly indicated (e.g., biopsy for a suspicious mass). The hoped-for participation in decision making can still occur prior to major treatment interventions that the patient should be attending to and passing on (e.g., risky surgical resection of a confirmed mass). Conversely, when the decision at hand involves important choices or trade-offs for the patient, or when similarly situated patients are known to choose differently, it would always seem appropriate to challenge a waiver (and, *equally,* more subtle inattentiveness) and advise the patient of the seriousness of the matters at hand. Equally, when patient compliance and self-monitoring are seen as clinically important factors, the waiving patient should be challenged. In all such situations, both the waiving patient *and* the inattentive one should be challenged and advised that there are matters that they must attend to personally.

In summary, the suggestion is that clinician response to patient waivers of informed consent (explicit or more subtle) should key to the goods and values of informed consent that may be voluntarily given up in the situation at hand. We might fruitfully return to the risk-benefit metaphor in this regard. The explicitly waiving patient should be queried as to what benefit he sees in not hearing the information, such as not being assaulted by facts that he is presently unable to bear. The clinician might then accept this or advise the patient of the risks of such behavior, such as not hearing information that he needs to for compliance or adaptive reasons.

The inattentive patient, for his part, will emerge in the third stage of the informed consent, when he is asked to repeat what he has just been told. Vague responses at such a juncture, particularly to the extent real choices or concerns are ingredient in the situation, can then be responded to with more detail from the clinician. Further, to the extent profound and personal decisions are at hand, the clinician should challenge any vague, seemingly inattentive responses, even to the point of giving the patient a short soliloquy on the need for patient participation in informed consent. As in the past, a major variable affecting the clinician's degree of response will concern where the patient is on the spectrum of treatments from those clearly indicated to those involving profound and personal choices. To the extent matters approach the latter extreme, the clinician should be increasingly resistant to patient waivers and, in extreme cases, simply not accept them. In this regard, what the law and the patient autonomy enthusiasts are comfortable with should often alarm the clinician instead.

THE THERAPEUTIC PRIVILEGE EXCEPTION

The basic justification of the therapeutic privilege exception is that in some special cases informed consent might itself seriously harm the patient and thus can be appropriately deleted or abbreviated. This exception appeals directly to the ancient "do no harm" injunction of medicine. In effect, the primary principles of beneficence and autonomy come into direct conflict with this exception.

As a legal matter, the sense of and conditions for this exception seem to vary enormously. Faden and Beauchamp portray the range of options well

> The precise formulation of the privilege varies widely among the jurisdictions. If framed broadly, it can permit physicians to withhold information if disclosure would cause *any* counter-therapeutic deterioration, however slight, in the physical, psychological or emotional condition of the patient. If framed narrowly, it can permit the physician to withhold information if and only if the

patient's knowledge of the information would have *serious* health-related consequences—for example, by jeopardizing the success of the treatment or harming the patient psychologically by critically impairing relevant decisionmaking processes. (Faden and Beauchamp, 1986, p. 37)

The options and applications at hand need sorting out. The possibility that disclosure might "critically impair decisionmaking processes" is essentially a form of the incompetence exception. A paradigm instance of this sense of the exception would be a presently stable but brittle psychiatric patient who might predictably decompensate as a direct result of disclosure (e.g., that he had a life-threatening malignancy). This would appear to be a cogent but extremely rare instance for the legitimate exercise of the exception. Another arguably legitimate use of the exception might arise with an anxious or agitated patient suffering from unstable angina. Disclosure might heighten agitation to the point that a lethal arrythmia might result.

But these two paradigm cases would seem to be more appropriately subsumed under other exceptions, incompetence for the former, the emergency exception for the latter. Neither gets us to the heart of the therapeutic exception, an exception based purely on the harm of disclosure to a patient, where there are arguably both time for this disclosure and a patient who appears to have sufficient competence to understand and respond to it.

To further focus on the real issue at hand, the therapeutic exception usually does not involve the tactic of eliminating informed consent altogether. Given an alert and oriented patient and the time for discussion, it would not be *tactically* feasible to say nothing at all to the patient about what is at hand and what is planned and simply impose treatment. Instead, the tactic is to delete certain harmful aspects of the usual informed consent, but still proceed with the attempt to get consent. The paradigm deletion here would be the fact that the patient has some form of cancer, and the appeal of the therapeutic exception would be that to disclose this to the patient would cause him serious psychological or emotional pain, that it would destroy the patient's remaining time, or make him very depressed. Other potential harms of such a disclosure that have been traditionally appealed to include that the patient might commit suicide or withdraw from care.

To frame the exception in this way allows it to have a very broad application. This is not a merely theoretical remark. Up until the last decade, this form of the exception was used widely and routinely to justify not disclosing life-threatening or terminal diagnoses to patients, paradigmatically the patient with cancer. Usually, I am informed by senior physicians, such a lack of disclosure was accompanied by false reassurance to the patient, disclosure was kept to a discussion of symptoms the patient was experiencing and what would be done to relieve them, and families regularly colluded wholeheartedly in the deception.

Such a widespread practice of deception is well documented and has been, in the last decade or so, roundly discredited. The classic work that elegantly sums up why this practice is inappropriate is Sissela Bok's book on *Lying*, specifically her chapter on "Lies to the Sick and Dying" (Bok, 1979, pp. 232–55). And part of the elegance of Bok's argument is that she meets the paternalistic physician on his own ground—namely, beneficence. Identifying numerous ways in which this practice itself tends to harm patients, Bok's ultimate argument is that, all things considered, such deception is likely to be more harmful to the patient than telling the truth. By depriving such a patient of the possibility of autonomous choice (itself a harm), such deception might lead to the patient's consenting to experimental or aggressive therapies that he would not otherwise accept. Bok further points out that such patients often still suspect something is wrong, may thus be afflicted by corrosive worry in spite of all physician assurances, could conclude matters are worse than they actually are, and will be deprived of the opportunity to accomplish last things, such as drawing up a will, saying good-bye, and so forth. Truth telling is thus essential to the push for death with dignity.

Bok and others have also noted the morally corrosive effect and burden placed on staff and families, particularly as they continue to manipulate or lie to the patient to keep the charade going, the inauthentic character of the patient's remaining time, and the exponentially deleterious effect of such behavior when participating family members themselves come in for treatment and are themselves reassured (perhaps appropriately) by their own physician in language strikingly like that previously offered to the deceived patient. It has also been repeatedly pointed out that such patients rarely commit suicide when told the truth, and a patient's decision to withdraw from treatment is now generally accepted as not only a reasonable outcome but often a prudent choice.

Along with these considerations, it is also now the case that with increasing patient awareness of cancer, such deceptions simply do not work for long, however skilled the deceivers. Patients are often themselves thinking about cancer or some life-threatening situation early on and will tend to ask about it. Even if they do not ask, they are often already worrying about it, so silence indicates nothing. This is probably also the case as so many families have recently been presented with the specter of a loved one with a terminal illness going through the "last rites" of medicine.

In the end, I submit, any broad exercise of this exception should be considered patently unethical. Even if we ignore the right of the patient to informed consent and autonomous choice, the exception is clearly offensive on beneficence grounds; in other words, it is highly likely to be more harmful to the patient than its alternative.

This leaves us with the possibility that the exception might be exercised in some narrower sense, most likely on the grounds of some special characteristic of the patient. A paradigm instance of this would be a patient whom the physician or family believes to be particularly prone to depression or other adverse psychological reactions if full disclosure is given. But, again, the previous harms of nondisclosure (or deception and lying) noted above are just as pertinent to this patient as to any other. Nor will it necessarily be any easier to carry off and sustain such a charade with this sort of patient. Also, that such a patient will, in fact, decompensate as a result of such a disclosure is highly conjectural before the fact, ignores the fact that depression is a natural response to such news, and is arguably more appropriately seen as a stage that therapy or counseling can assist the patient to work through. I would thus submit that even on a narrow interpretation of the exception, it should be received with the greatest skepticism, and it lacks any credible account of its justifying principles and conditions.

SUMMARY REMARKS

The approach to these three exceptions, as well as to that of the exception based on patient incompetence, has been essentially guided by the fact that informed consent and patient participation in decision making are important activities and should be deleted only for clear and strong reasons. We found these to be absent in the case of the traditional exception based on therapeutic privilege. As to the waiver exception, we noted various reasons to greet such a response with skepticism but, given the fact that many patients seem to exercise this option *sub rosa*, embraced the idea that such waivers, explicit or not, should only be challenged if significant informative or decision making tasks would thus be deleted. The emergency exception, for its part, was left mainly to objective medical judgment as to the disvalue associated with pausing for informed consent, and options such as abbreviated consents were generally disparaged as of little significance.

Our final task in this volume lies in summarizing the course of our discussion and its findings. This will be accomplished by reflecting on the enterprise of informed consent.

9

Concluding Remarks

By way of conclusion, we need to accomplish three final tasks: (1) provide a basic summary of the argument of this work; (2) make one final point regarding the clinical variables and variable responses that our informed consent intervention must key to, offered under the heading of "the clinician's discretion"; and (3) place this intervention within the broader context of clinician communications with patients.

THE BASIC ARGUMENT OF THIS WORK

Our aim has been to develop a sense of informed consent as a useful tool for medical management, an intervention that would change outcomes at the bedside for the better. In chapter 1, we found that the law offered no such implement, focused as it was for all its rhetoric on the ways that tort law might identify actionable departures from minimally adequate informed consents. Whatever minimal goals the law legitimately chose to pursue, it was simply not adequate to the ethical and clinical goods and values that were at stake. Moreover, the law proceeded in terms of a presumption regarding competence and a "bits and pieces" sense of understanding that did not reflect the actual capacities or needs of patients in the situation of illness, nor did it reflect the ways in which such factors varied from situation to situation and patient to patient. Finally, even if one accepted the narrower focus of the law's approach, it failed to provide sufficient operational guidance to determine how to satisfy its requirements—for example, in its standards for disclosure or for the assessment of competence.

The "new ethos of patient autonomy" fared no better, as chapter 2 documents. Along with presuming competence in most patients, with little recognition of or provision for its common diminishments, it proceeded on the basis of a self-stultifying adversarial view of the

relationship between physician and patient. The relation was charac-
terized as that of moral strangers, who were unlikely to share or
understand each other's values. The resolution for this deficiency
came in the form of the notion of "freedom from interference"—in
effect, that if only physicians would stop paternalizing their patients
and provide them with sufficient information, patient autonomy
would blossom forth. We disagreed with this vision, however, noting
that it proceeded in terms of an impoverished sense of freedom with
regard, for example, to the counseling and adaptive needs many
patients have. Such a view was also seen as flawed because it did not
recognize that the active assistance of the clinician is often indispens-
able to patient autonomy, not just in its decision-making activity but
also in its need for protection and enhancement. We also refused to
allow the proponents of patient autonomy to use the trump of freedom to ground their essentially one-dimensional sense of patient
autonomy—as mainly a decision-making enterprise leavened by some
inchoate choice—and agreed to take up the paternalist's gauntlet
regarding what goods and values are actually at stake in the consent
situation.

We then came to the unsettling conclusion that, as the goods and
values informed consent might pursue came into clearer relief (per
chapter 4), the possibility that it might successfully pursue them had
become markedly less likely (per chapter 3). Aside from the marginal
results of most empirical studies and clinicians' common experience of
patients, heightened skepticism arose from further reflection on the
presence of diminished competence in illness, the numerous barriers
to autonomy in the situation of illness, and the complexities ingredient in medical decision making itself. But, conversely, as this skepticism increased, the sense and importance of the various goods and
values that were at stake did also, so we found that we did not have
the option of siding with the "myth of informed consent" crowd.

Our response to this impasse was to conceive of the problem of
informed consent as a Gordian knot that would be unlikely to admit
of any intellectual unraveling. In chapter 5, we elected instead to
sever it by the provision of a detailed operational model of informed
consent where the various goods and values that informed consent
might capture would be given their due for the most part. We elected
to invest our effort primarily in a discrete event model of informed
consent. This model was retailed in our chapter 6. Certain already recognized goods and values were to be provided for within this model:

the authorization by the patient to proceed, a rule-out for hesitation, ambivalence, and misconceptions on the patient's part, the need for some core disclosure of the essential choice at hand over and above the details, and a feedback mechanism where the patient's level of understanding, at the level of the core disclosure, could be assessed and enhanced as desired or needed. Other goods and values were treated as variables that might or might not be involved, depending on the patient's situation and prospects, needs and capacities. Detailed actual understanding, the basic focus of many other accounts, was treated as a good that might or might not be important depending on the situation at hand, the patient's capacity for and level of interest in appreciating the details, and the clinician's perception of the need for such detailed insight. In effect, we accepted the idea that a detailed actual understanding might not be necessary for an adequate informed consent, allowing the patient to determine the level of detail and insight he wanted, at least in the more common cases where the treatment was seen as clearly indicated by the clinician. The clinician, however, was also held responsible to recognize when some basic level of actual understanding was important, as when important personal decisions were at hand, compliance and cooperation needed shoring up, or counseling and values clarification were indicated.

Having provided the event model of informed consent in detail, in chapter 7 we then proceeded to reflect on the notion of competence, particularly in the sense of when we might be triggered to assess it further rather than typically assuming its presence, as the law recommends. In our treatment of competence we relegated factors that many tend to see as part of an assessment of competence to mere triggers for an assessment that does not itself include them, such as unfavorable decisions by patients or the presence of mental illness. Equally, we ended up strongly committed to maintaining the status of competence for patients by insisting, first, that an attempt be made to remove such triggering factors, and then, whether or not they are removed, that there be an attempt to assist the patient to credibly participate in the specific decision-making task at hand. In the end, our account should be received as being as extreme as any in its concern to respect, protect, and strive to enhance patient autonomy.

Chapter 8 then finished the explication of our model by evaluating the three main exceptions to informed consent for competent patients. The emergency exception, based on objective medical criteria, was mainly left intact, though we did leaven it with concerns about how it could come to destroy the rule. We also noted that a preventive ethics approach to anticipatable crises was markedly preferable. The waiver exception, for its part, was seen as a more explicit and candid form of the commonly seen behavior of the inattentive patient, and both were accepted as legitimate choices that an autonomous individual could make. We still criticized both types of waiver as unacceptable when important choices were at hand for the patient, or a detailed knowledge by the patient was important for compliance and self-monitoring, as well as for counseling and adaptive purposes in more extreme situations of chronic and terminal illness. Finally, the traditional exception based on therapeutic privilege was essentially ruled out of court as being wholly contrary to the thrust of our enterprise and lacking any cogent example or account.

THE CLINICIAN'S DISCRETION

Having said all this, we need to face one final issue here. There are various ways to express it, but perhaps its most forceful form would come if we imagine some overworked clinician, having navigated through the preceding, asking the following question: "This is all very well and good, but there appear to be so many variables here, and so few minutes during the day, that I am left to wonder (and worry) how I will know in any particular instance whether I have satisfied the demands of your model. In short, when am I done?" This clinician might continue: "I notice that you have prudently recognized that many patients are not comfortable with or do not desire a decision-making role, and more than a few really do not listen to the details. Rather, they are waiting for my recommendation and usually accept it. I note further that you allow for the stages of your model to key to such realities somewhat. At least in your third stage of 'assessment, clarification, and patient choice,' you note that the content of this stage will mainly be determined by the patient, and given that some patients will have very little to say or ask here, I gather I can accept the patient who simply says, 'Do what you think is best, Doc,' without requiring that he perform further. Similarly, in the previous two stages where I am retailing the details, I would somehow assume that you would allow me to gauge my presentation to the educational and linguistic level of the patient, so the informed consent for the same exact intervention may well vary significantly from patient to patient.

But I note elsewhere—for example, in your discussion of the waiver exception in the previous chapter—that you think I may need to prod some patients to higher levels of understanding than they tend to want if the decision is significantly value-charged. All this makes some sense, and sounds like you are trying to key to clinical realities, but it also appears to be byzantine in its possibilities, which is to say unrealistic given the time usually available. Or, more simply, I am left worrying that whatever the problems with the law, at least I believe I have some sense as to when I have satisfied its demands. With your model, I am left unsure."

This query requires a final discussion here, particularly regarding the sort of judgment calls that a clinician would have to make within this model. And the issue here is best met, I submit, by referring again to the work of Howard Brody, specifically to the argument of his book *The Healer's Power*. In this work, Brody's central argument is that medical ethics is about power and its responsible use (Brody, 1992, p. 12). Feeling that much of medical ethics is flawed because it ignores or otherwise submerges the power aspect of medical care, he insists, "Physicians have considerable power to alter the course of illness. . . . The problem is to empower physicians for the performance of their essential tasks while protecting the patient from the potential misuses and abuses of power" (Brody, 1992, p. 36). Concurring with this claim in general, I would first make the point that although the term "power" seems apt when Brody is discussing ethical issues like the placebo effect, I much prefer the term "discretion" in the current context. To the main point, however, in Brody's "transparency" model of informed consent, as well as the one advocated in this work, there are numerous points at which the clinician will need to make "judgment calls"—that is, exercise discretion—somehow guided by the "spirit" of the model. And a summary of some of the basic similarities and differences between the two models should go far to respond to this last thorny issue of clinician discretion. In effect, though the two models agree in many ways, I see Brody's approach as interestingly wrong in a number of senses but concur absolutely with his challenge that the issue of the clinician's power (or discretion) is a central issue here.

The models agree on a number of basic points, such as the presence of diminished competence in many patients, the presence of numerous barriers to effective communication and understanding, and the fact that many patients lack interest in the details (or even if they desire understanding, still do not want to assume a primary decision-making role). Second, the models agree (and arise) out of a common conviction that the silent world of doctor and patient needs to be reformed, but further agree that neither the law nor what I call the "new ethos of patient autonomy" provides an adequate or effective reformation.

Brody's transparency model further recommends (1) that the ground on which disclosure rests is the clinician's own thought processes as he proceeds to the point of making a recommendation for the patient, and (2) that the clinician must exercise discretion regarding numerous issues, including how the information will be framed, how specific the disclosure will be, and, crucially, when the clinician is finished, all keyed to variations in the patient's ability, interest, and needs in understanding.

Now to key disclosure to the clinician's own thought processes is clear guidance and would seem to be generally adequate; as Brody says, the physician merely needs to think out loud for the patient. Equally, we have already accepted the idea that the form and content of disclosure, as well as its timing, should key to the patient's capacities, interests, and needs. But, at least as a question of emphasis (Brody might well agree with what follows), Brody seems to keep his model more clinician-centered than is indicated.

That is, it seems that once the clinician has rendered his thought processes explicit for the patient, and whatever questions the patient has have been satisfactorily answered, the clinician can decide that he is finished. But we must demur here. In the majority of cases, where the treatment is clearly indicated, we agree. But we have also chosen to emphasize that other variables may well be present (per chapter 4). Here, for all Brody seems to say, once the clinician has been "transparent" to the patient, and the patient indicates he is satisfied (a vague nod might suffice), it appears that the "conversation" is done.

But it may not be, as we have previously argued in detail. The inattentive patient may need to be stimulated, against his own tendency, to better appreciate what is in the offing for all those reasons we initially identified—for example, that important, value-charged issues are at hand, compliance and self-monitoring may be pivotal to clinical success, or the issue of competence may have been triggered. On any of these grounds, all potentially crucial components of prudent medical management, further efforts, beyond what the clinician finds clinically significant or the patient wants to hear, may be necessary. For precisely such reasons, the third feedback stage, which Brody does not formally incorporate, was built into our model.

At one point, but at least with insufficient emphasis for our purposes, Brody seems to envision that the physician may well prod the patient to reflect further than either of them personally had tended to do. As he says, the clinician may at times "cut a discussion short because she judges that all that is necessary has been done. But she will be just as likely to draw the conversation out further by quizzing the patient on whether he has reflected carefully on what he has just been told" (Brody, 1992, p. 107). But aside from not formally emphasizing the latter tactic in his model, Brody provides no sense as to when such prodding should occur.

In sum, we should accept the variability (and thus discretion) commended here but, in the same breath, presume to take Brody to task as he generally does not make such an emphasis when formally stating his model. It seems to be satisfied with what might well remain, in any situation, a one-way communication, from physician to patient. As he himself notes in passing, this will occasionally be inadequate to the tasks and needs at hand. In sum, there will probably be little or no difference between the two models in the majority of medical interventions. We should embrace Brody's transparency model as a needed and generally adequate reformation, but, as stated, it appears liable to be too one-sided or physician-directed in a minority of cases.

By way of concluding summary regarding such discretion, this might all be expressed in another fashion. Brody's transparency model surely goes far to answer the clinician's question that started this section—when do I know when I am done? The answer "once you have made your own thought processes regarding the case transparent to the patient" surely offers a standard that any clinician can easily key to. And clinician discretion can then justify itself in this ground usually, but with the additional proviso that further interactive conversations may be needed when the additional concerns and values highlighted in chapter 4 are also at stake. This said, however, a query from a quite different quarter merits response. The "patient autonomy" advocate may well express some real misgivings at this juncture, especially regarding the discretion that Brody and I want to allow for. Our response here takes us, in effect, back to the initial purposes and driving forces of this work. In sum, given that the legal version of informed consent is just not adequate to the purposes at hand, a model emphasizing the clinical good and values that informed consent may need to address is the only resort for those who actually want to reform medical practice and change outcomes for the better. But the point is that once one approaches all this clinically, these goods and values must be seen as only occasionally and variably present. And thus it is bootless to call for some universal response to them when they are often not significantly at stake. In sum, once we try to rectify matters by taking the paternalist's challenge seriously, we end up with capacities, interests, and needs that vary considerably from patient to patient and case to case. And only by allowing for clinician discretion regarding all this can we earn the credibility that may actually motivate clinicians to embrace this model.

TALKING TO PATIENTS

A few final remarks merit making by way of conclusion of this discussion. We should first note that this discussion does not speak to certain important features of the informed consent enterprise. For one thing, there is a wealth of information in the clinical literature on tactics that enhance communication and patient insight. This especially tactical literature is enormous and is particularly found in writings regarding malpractice prophylaxis and how to enhance patient compliance and satisfaction, as well as in a whole genre of writings regarding how to communicate effectively with patients. Eric Cassell's two-volume work *Talking with Patients* is strongly recommended to the reader in this regard (Cassell, 1985).

Second, both for training the neophyte and for the sake of having a standard of practice to appeal to, the construction of standard informed consents for specific procedures, especially on the level of the comprehensive and core disclosure stages of our model, is needed. Here, to refer to Howard Brody one last time, do not believe that a wholly physician-centered standard for disclosure will necessarily be adequate for legal protection, and thus do not see the comprehensive disclosure stage as collapsing into some core transparency stage. As suggested previously, clinicians should refer to legal authorities in their particular jurisdictions in this regard. The construction of such forms is, of course, a job for those who provide such treatments, but it should be noted that the interactive model provided here should assist such a process. That is, given a clinician who is sufficiently aware of the risks, benefits, and limitations of a procedure to legitimately offer it to a patient, this model should provide a vehicle to test and further enhance any such formulation. As such stock presentations are offered to individual patients, problems of patient comprehension and satisfaction should emerge both during and after the event that will help instruct the clinician as to what form of presentation is the most efficient and effective. As the silence at the bedside is replaced by mutual exploration and discussion, patients' concerns and fears should become more apparent to clinicians, and can be formally anticipated, rather than be allowed to fester unnoted and cause trouble later. Equally, I would expect the realm wherein similarly situated patients might decide differently—those cases that are truly value-charged— both to become clearer and to expand, not only to the extent that they are assisted to attain greater insight in individual situations but to the extent that such idiosyncratic concerns and differences are actively solicited.

I would finally hope that the vision of the physician-patient interaction advocated here is not seen by clinicians as just efficient and effective but also attractive. The informed consent intervention need not be seen as an unrealistic foreign body foisted on medicine by outsiders who neither understand the realities within which the care of the patient is pursued nor trust those who have dedicated their lives to providing it. Rather, it is portrayed as one more way in which clinicians can aid their patients and satisfy their needs. As promised, we are talking about the provision of good medical care, no more and no less.

References and Suggested Readings

Abernethy, V. 1984. Compassion, control, and decisions about competency. *American Journal of Psychiatry* 141: 53–58.

Abernethy, V., and K. Lundin. 1980. Patient competence: Conditions for giving or withholding consent. In *Frontiers in medical ethics*, edited by V. Abernethy, 79–98. Cambridge: Ballinger.

Ackerman, T.F. 1982. Why doctors should intervene. *Hastings Center Report* 12: 14–17.

Agich, G. 1990. Reassessing autonomy in long-term care. *Hastings Center Report* 20: 12–17.

Alfidi, R.J. 1971. Informed consent: A study of patient reaction. *Journal of the American Medical Association* 216: 1325.

———. 1975. Controversy, alternatives and decisions in complying with the legal doctrine of informed consent. *Radiology* 114: 231–34.

Andrews, L.B. 1984. Informed consent status and the decision-making process. *Journal of Legal Medicine* 52:163–217.

Annas, G.J. 1975. *The rights of hospital patients*. New York: Avon Books.

———. 1976. Avoiding malpractice suits through the use of informed consent. *Current Problems of Pediatrics* 6: 3–48.

———. 1994. Informed consent, cancer, and truth in prognosis. *New England Journal of Medicine* 330: 223–25.

Appelbaum, P.S. and L.H. Roth. 1981. Empirical assessment of competency to consent to psychiatric hospitalization. *American Journal of Psychiatry* 138: 1170–76.

Appelbaum, P.S., C.W. Lidz, and A. Meisel. 1987. *Informed consent: Legal theory and clinical practice*. New York: Oxford University Press.

Appelbaum, P.S., and L.H. Roth. 1981. Clinical issues in the assessment of competency. *American Journal of Psychiatry* 138: 1462–67.

Appelbaum, P.S., and T.G. Gutheil. 1980. "Rotting with their rights on": Constitutional theory and clinical reality in drug refusal by psychiatric patients. *Bulletin American Academy of Psychiatry and Law* 7: 306–15.

Balint, J., and W. Shelton. 1996. Regaining the initiative: Forging a new model of the patient-physician relationship. *Journal of the American Medical Association* 275: 887–91.

Barbour, G.L., and M.J. Blumenkrantz. 1978. Videotape aids informed consent decision. *Journal of the American Medical Association* 240: 2741–42.

Baron, C. 1987. On knowing one's chains and decking them with flowers: Limits on patient autonomy in "The Silent World of Doctor and Patient." *Western New England Law Review* 9: 31–41.

Baumgarten, E. 1980. The concept of competence in medical ethics. *Journal of Medical Ethics* 6: 180–84.

Beauchamp, T.L., and J.F. Childress. 1989. *Principles of biomedical ethics*. 3d ed. New York: Oxford University Press.

Beauchamp, T.L., and L.B. McCullough. 1984. *Medical ethics: The moral responsibilities of physicians*. Englewood Cliffs, N.J.: Prentice Hall.

Bedell, S.E., and T.L. Delbanco. 1984. Choices about cardiopulmonary resuscitation in the hospital. *New England Journal of Medicine* 310: 1089–92.

Beecher, H.K. 1955. The powerful placebo. *Journal of the American Medical Association* 159: 1602–06.

————. 1966. Ethics and clinical research. *New England Journal of Medicine* 274: 1354–60.

Bengler, J.H., C. Pennington, M. Metcalfe, and E. Freis. 1980. Informed consent: How much does the patient understand? *Clinical Pharmacology and Therapeutics* 27: 435–40.

Benson, H., and D.P. McCallie. 1979. Angina pectoris and the placebo effect. *New England Journal of Medicine* 300: 1424–29.

Bergen, R.P. 1974. The confusing law of informed consent. *Journal of the American Medical Association* 229: 325.

Bergman, M., S.B. Akin, and P. Felig. 1990. Understanding the diabetic patient from a psychological dimension: Implications for the patient and the provider. *American Journal of Psychoanalysis* 50 (1): 25–33.

Biros, M.H. et al. 1995. Informed consent in emergency research: Consensus statement from the coalition conference of acute resuscitation and critical care researchers. *Journal of the American Medical Association* 273 (16): 1283–87.

Blanchard, C.G. et al. 1990. Physician behaviors, patient perceptions, and patient characteristics as predictors of satisfaction of hospitalized adult cancer patients. *Cancer* 65: 186–92.

Blanchard, C.G., J.C. Ruckdeschel, E.B. Blanchard et al. 1983. Interactions between oncologists and patients during rounds. *Annals of Internal Medicine* 99: 694–99.

Blustein, J. 1993. The family in medical decisionmaking. *Hastings Center Report* 23: 6–13.

Boisaubin, E.V., and R. Dresser. 1987. Informed consent in emergency care: Illusion and reform. *Annals of Emergency Medicine* 16 (1): 62–67.

Bok, S. 1978. *Lying: Moral choice in public and private life*. New York: Vintage Books.

Botkin, J.R. 1989. Informed consent for lumbar puncture. *American Journal of Diseases of Children* 143 (8): 899–904.

Brett, A.S. 1981. Hidden ethical issues in clinical decision analysis. *New England Journal of Medicine* 305: 1150–53.

Brett, A.S., and L.B. McCullough. 1986. When patients request specific interventions: Defining the limits of the physician's obligation. *New England Journal of Medicine* 315: 1347–51.

Brock, D.W. 1991. The ideal of shared decision making between physicians and patients. *Kennedy Institute of Ethics Journal* 11: 28–47.

Brock, D., and S. Wartman. 1990. When competent patients make irrational choices. *New England Journal of Medicine* 322: 1595–99.

Brody, D.S. 1980. The patient's role in clinical decision-making. *Annals of Internal Medicine* 93: 718–22.

Brody, H. 1980 *Placebos and the philosophy of medicine*. Chicago: University of Chicago Press.

———. 1982. The lie that heals: The ethics of giving placebos. *Annals of Internal Medicine* 97: 112–18.

———. 1983. Ethics in family medicine: Patient autonomy and the family unit. *Journal of Family Practice* 17: 975.

———. 1985. Autonomy revisited: Progress in medical ethics. *Journal of the Royal Society of Medicine* 78: 380–87.

———. 1987. *Stories of sickness*. New Haven: Yale University Press.

———. 1989. Transparency: Informed consent in primary care. *Hastings Center Report* 19: 5–9.

———. 1992. *The Healer's Power*. New Haven: Yale University Press.

Brown, P. 1986. Psychiatric treatment refusal, patient competence, and informed consent. *International Journal of Law and Psychiatry* 8: 94.

Buchanan, A. 1978. Medical paternalism. *Philosophy and Public Affairs* 7: 370–90.

Buchanan, A.E., and D.W. Brock. 1989. *Deciding for others: The ethics of surrogate decisionmaking*. New York: Cambridge University Press.

Burt, R.A. 1979. *Taking care of strangers: The rule of law in doctor-patient relations*. New York: Free Press.

Cairns, J.A. 1985. Aspirin, sulfinpyrazone, or both in unstable angina. *New England Journal of Medicine* 313: 1369–75.

Callahan, D. 1984. Autonomy: A moral good, not a moral obsession. *Hastings Center Report* 14: 40–42.

Caplan, A.L. 1988. Informed consent and provider-patient relationships in rehabilitation medicine. *Archives of Medical Rehabilitation* 69: 312–17.

———. 1995. Review of Stephen Wear's *Informed consent: Patient autonomy and physician beneficence in clinical medicine*. *Journal of the American Geriatrics Association* 43 (12): 3–5.

Capron, A.M. 1974. Informed consent in catastrophic disease research and treatment. *University of Pennsylvania Law Review* 123: 340–438.

———. 1993. Duty, truth, and whole human beings. *Hastings Center Report* 23: 13–14.

Carney, B. 1987. Bone marrow transplant: Nurses' and physicians' perceptions of informed consent. *Cancer Nursing* 10 (5): 252–59.

Cassell, E.J. 1976. *The healer's art: A new approach to the doctor-patient relationship*. Philadelphia: J. B. Lippincott.

————. 1977. The function of medicine. *Hastings Center Report* 7: 16–19.

————. 1982. The nature of suffering and the goals of medicine. *New England Journal of Medicine* 306: 639–45.

————. 1985a. *Talking with patients*. Vol. 1, *The theory of doctor-patient communication*. Cambridge, Mass.: MIT Press.

————. 1985b. *Talking with patients*. Vol. 2, *Clinical techniques*. Cambridge, Mass.: MIT Press.

Cassileth, B.R., R.V. Zupkis, K. Sutton-Smith, and V. March. 1980. Informed consent: Why are its goals imperfectly realized? *New England Journal of Medicine* 302: 896–900.

Childress, J. 1982. *Who should decide?* New York: Oxford University Press.

————. 1990. The place of autonomy in bioethics. *Hastings Center Report* 20: 12–16.

Childress, J., and M.D. Siegler. 1984. Metaphors and models of doctor-patient relationships: Their implications for autonomy. *Theoretical Medicine* 5: 17–29.

Clark, J.A., D.A. Potter, and J.B. McKinlay. 1991. Bringing social structure back into the clinical decision making. *Social Science and Medicine* 32: 853–66.

Comstock, L., E. Hooper, J. Goodwin, and J. Goodwin. 1982. Physician behaviors that correlate with patient satisfaction. *Journal of Medical Education* 57: 105–12.

Consumer Reports. 1994. Yonkers, N.Y.: Consumers Union of United States.

Cousins, N. 1982. The physician as communicator. *Journal of the American Medical Association* 248: 587–89.

Crowden, A. 1996. Review of Stephen Wear's *Informed consent: Patient autonomy and physician beneficence in clinical medicine*. *Bioethics* 10 (1): 83–86.

Culver, C.M., R.B. Ferrel, and R.M. Green. 1980. ECT and special problems of informed consent. *American Journal of Psychiatry* 137: 586–91.

Culver, C.M., and B. Gert. 1982. *Philosophy in medicine: Conceptual and ethical issues in medicine and psychiatry*. New York: Oxford University Press.

Cutter, M.A.G., and E.E. Shelp, eds. 1991. *Competency: A study of informal competency determinations in primary care*. Dordrecht, Netherlands: Kluwer Academic Publishers.

Denney, M.K., D. Williamson, and R. Penn. 1975. Informed consent: Emotional responses of patients. *Postgraduate Medicine* 60: 205–9.

Depaulo, B.M., and R. Rosenthal. 1979. Ambivalence, discrepancy, and deception in nonverbal communication. In *Skill in nonverbal communication: Individual differences*, edited by R. Rosenthal, 204–48. Cambridge, Mass.: Oelgeschlager, Gunn, and Hain.

Donnelly, W. 1988. Righting the medical record: Transforming chronicle into story. *Journal of the American Medical Association* 260 (6): 823–25.

Doukas, D.J., and L.B. McCullough. 1991. The values history. *Journal of Family Practice* 32: 145–50.

Drane, J.F. 1984. Competency to give informed consent. *Journal of the American Medical Association* 252: 925–27.

————. 1985. The many faces of competency. *Hastings Center Report* 15: 17–21.

————. 1988. *Becoming a good doctor: The place of virtue and character in medical ethics.* St. Louis, Mo.: Sheed & Ward.

Duff, R.S. 1988. Unshared and shared decisionmaking: Reflections on helplessness and healing. In *The physician as captain of the ship: A critical reappraisal,* edited by N. M. P. King, L. R. Churchill, and A. W. Cross, 191–222. Dordrecht, Netherlands: Reidel.

Eisenberg, J.M. 1979. Sociologic influences on decision-making by clinicians. *Annals of Internal Medicine* 90: 233–56.

Elfant, A.B., C. Korn, L. Mendez et al. 1995. Recall of informed consent after endoscopic procedures. *Diseases of the Colon and Rectum* 38: 1–3.

Emanuel, E.J., and N.N. Dubler. 1993. Preserving the physician-patient relationship in the era of managed care. *Journal of the American Medical Association* 273: 323–29.

Emanuel, E.J., and L.L. Emanuel. 1992. Four models of the physician-patient relationship. *Journal of the American Medical Association* 267: 2221–26.

Engel, G.L. 1977. The need for a new medical model. *Science* 196: 129–36.

————. 1978. The biopsychosocial model and the education of health professionals. *Annals of the New York Academy of Sciences* 310: 169–81.

————. 1980. The clinical application of the biopsychosocial model. *American Journal of Psychiatry* 137: 535–44.

Engelhardt, H.T. 1982. Bioethics in pluralistic societies. *Perspectives in Biology and Medicine* 26: 64–77.

————. 1986. *The foundations of bioethics.* New York: Oxford University Press.

Engelhardt, H.T., and M.A. Rie. 1988. Morality for the medical industrial complex. *New England Journal of Medicine* 319: 1086–89.

Epstein, L.C., and L. Lasagna. 1969. Obtaining informed consent: Form or substance. *Archives of Internal Medicine* 123: 682.

Faden, R. 1977. Disclosure and informed consent: Does it matter how we tell it? *Health Education Monographs* 5: 198–215.

Faden, R., and T. Beauchamp. 1980. Decision-making and informed consent. *Social Indicators Research* 7: 313–36.

Faden, R., and A. Faden. 1977. False belief and the refusal of medical treatment. *Journal of Medical Ethics* 3: 133–36.

————. 1978. Informed consent in medical practice: With particular reference to neurology. *Archives of Neurology* 35: 761–64.

————. 1986. *A history and theory of informed consent.* New York: Oxford University Press.

Faden, R. et al. 1981. Disclosure standards and informed consent. *Journal of Health, Politics, Policy and Law* 6: 255–84.

Feinberg, J. 1971. Legal paternalism. *Canadian Journal of Philosophy* 1: 105–24.

Fellner, C.H., and J.R. Marshall. 1970. Kidney donors—the myth of informed consent. *American Journal of Psychiatry* 126: 1245–51.

Ferrell, R. et al. 1984. Volitional disability and physician attitudes toward noncompliance. *The Journal of Medicine and Philosophy* 9 (4): 333–51.

Final Report of the Tuskegee Syphilis Study Ad Hoc Advisory Panel. 1977. In *Ethics in medicine,* edited by J. Reiser et al., 316–21. Cambridge, Mass.: MIT Press.

Finkelstein, D., M.K. Smith, and R. Faden. 1993. Informed consent and medical ethics. *Archives of Ophthalmology* 111 (3): 324–26.

Fisher, R., and W. Ury. 1981. *Getting to yes: Negotiating agreement without giving in.* Boston: Houghton-Mifflin.

Fisher, S., and T.D. Alexandra, eds. 1983. *The social organization of doctor-patient communication.* Washington, D.C.: Center for Applied Linguistics.

Fisher, W.R. 1987. *Human communication as narration: Toward a philosophy of reason, value, and action.* Columbia, S.C.: University of South Carolina Press.

Freedman, B. 1975. A moral theory of informed consent. *Hastings Center Report* 54: 32–39.

———. Competence, marginal and otherwise. *International Journal of Law and Psychiatry* 4: 53–72.

Freeman, W.R., A.D. Pichard, and H. Smith. 1981. Effect of informed consent and educational background on patient knowledge, anxiety, and subjective responses to cardiac catheterization. *Catheterization and Cardiovascular Disease* 7: 119–34.

Friedlander, W.J. 1995. The evolution of informed consent in American medicine. *Perspectives in Biology and Medicine* 38: 499–510.

Fries, J.F., and E.F. Loftus. 1979. Informed consent: Right or rite? *CA-A Cancer Journal for Clinicians* 29: 316–18.

Gadow, S. 1980. Existential advocacy: Philosophic foundation of nursing. In *Nursing: Images and ideals: Opening dialogue with the humanities,* edited by S.F. Spickler and S. Gallow, 79–101. New York: Springer.

Gaylin, W. 1982. The competence of children: No longer all or none. *Hastings Center Report* 12: 33–38.

Gert, B., and C. Culver. 1981. Competence to consent: A philosophical overview. In *Competency and informed consent,* edited by N. Reating, 12–31. Rockville, Md.: National Institutes of Mental Health.

Gilligan, C. 1982. *In a different voice: Psychological theory and women's development.* Cambridge, Mass.: Harvard University Press.

Gold, J.A. 1993. Informed consent. *Archives of Ophthalmology* 111: 321–23.

Goldworth, A. 1996. Informed consent revisited. *Cambridge Quarterly of Healthcare Ethics* 5: 214–20.

Gorovitz, S. 1982. *Doctors' dilemmas: Moral conflict and medical care.* New York: Macmillan.

Gostin, L.O. 1995. Informed consent, cultural sensitivity, and respect for persons. *Journal of the American Medical Association* 274: 844–85.

Grundner, T.M. 1980. On the readability of surgical consent forms. *New England Journal of Medicine* 302: 900–902.

Gutheil, T.G., H. Burzstajn, and A. Brodsky. 1984. Malpractice prevention through the sharing of uncertainty: Informed consent and the therapeutic alliance. *New England Journal of Medicine* 311: 49–51.

Hackett, T.P., and N.H. Cassem. 1974. Development of a quantitative rating scale to assess denial. *Journal of Psychosomatic Research* 18: 93–100.

Hahn, R.A. 1982. Culture and informed consent: An anthropological perspective. In *Making health care decisions: The ethical and legal implications of informed consent in the patient-practitioner relationship.* Vol. 2. Washington,

D.C.: U.S. President's Commission for the Study of Ethical Problems in Medicine and Biomedical and Behavioral Research.

Hall, J.A., A.M. Epstein, M.L. DeCiantis, and B.J. McNeil. 1983. Physicians' liking for their patients: More evidence for the role of affect in medical care. *Health Psychology* 12: 140–46.

Hall, J.A., J.T. Irish, D.L. Roter et al. 1994. Gender in medical encounters: An analysis of physician and patient communication in a primary care setting. *Health Psychology* 13: 384–92.

Harris, L., and Associates. 1982. Views of informed consent and decision making: Parallel surveys of physicians and the public. In *Making health care decisions*. Vol. 2, 17–316. Washington, D.C.: U.S. President's Commission for the Study of Ethical Problems in Medicine and Biomedical and Behavioral Research.

Hilfiker, D. 1985. *Healing the wounds*. New York: Pantheon Books.

Holder, A. 1970. Informed consent: Its evolution. *Journal of the American Medical Association* 214: 1181–82.

Hudson, T. 1991. Informed consent problems become more complicated. *Hospitals* 65: 38–40.

Hull, R. 1978. Patients' rights and responsibilities: Questions of consent. In *Matters of life and death*, edited by J.E. Thomas, 277–97. Toronto: Samuel Stevens.

Hunter, K.M. 1991. *Doctors' stories: The narrative structure of medical knowledge*. Princeton, N J : Princeton University Press.

Hutson, M.M., and D. Blaha. 1991. Patients' recall of preoperative instruction for informed consent for an operation. *Journal of Bone and Joint Surgery* 73: 160–62.

Inglefinger, F.J. 1982. Informed (but uneducated) consent. *New England Journal of Medicine* 287: 465–66.

Inui, T.S., and W.B. Carter. 1985. Problems and prospects for health services research on provider-patient communication. *Medical Care* 23: 521–38.

Jackson, D.L., and S. Youngner. 1979. Patient autonomy and death with dignity. *New England Journal of Medicine* 301: 404–8.

Jakobovits, I. 1975. *Jewish medical ethics*. New York: Bloch.

James, D.H., and T.F. Ackerman. 1984. Patterns of primary care that create dependency. *American Journal of Diseases of Children* 138: 530–35.

Johnson, P.R. 1986. Patient autonomy in decision making: Recent trends in medical ethics. *Linacre Quarterly* 53 (2): 37–46.

Johnson, R.F. 1973. Consent in the emergency room. In *Legal medicine annual*, edited by C. Wecht, 345–56. New York: Appleton-Century-Crofts.

Jonsen, A.R., M. Siegler, and W.J. Winslade. 1982. *Clinical ethics*. New York: Macmillan.

Jonsen, A.R., and S. Toulmin. 1988. *The abuse of casuistry: A history of moral reasoning*. Berkeley: University of California Press.

Kaplan, S.H., S. Greenfield, and J.E. Ware. 1989. Assessing the effects of physician-patient interactions on the outcomes of chronic disease. *Medical Care* 27: 110–27.

Kapp, Marshall B. 1989. Enforcing patient preferences: Linking payment for medical care to informed consent. *Journal of the American Medical Association* 261: 1935–38.

Katz, J. 1981. Disclosure and consent in psychiatric practice. In *Law and ethics in the practice of psychiatry*, edited by C.K. Hofling, 91–117. New York: Brunner/Mazel.

———. 1984. *The silent world of the doctor and patient*. New York: Free Press.

Kelley, W.D., and S.R. Friesen. 1950. Do cancer patients want to be told? *Surgery* 27: 822–26.

King, N.M.P. 1991. *Making sense of advanced directives*. Dordrecht, Netherlands: Kluwer Academic Publishers.

Kleinman, A. 1988. *The illness narratives: Suffering, healing, and the human condition*. New York: Basic Books.

Knight, J. 1977. Judging competence: When the psychiatrist need, or need not, be involved. *Hastings Center Report* 7: 19–20.

Kodish, E., and S.G. Post. 1995. Oncology and hope. *Journal of Clinical Oncology* 13 (7): 1817–22.

Komrad, M. 1983. A defense of medical paternalism: Maximizing patients' autonomy. *Journal of Medical Ethics* 9: 38–44.

Kopelman, L.M. 1990. On the evaluative nature of competency and capacity judgments. *International Journal of Law and Psychiatry* 13 (4): 309–29.

Korsch, B.M., and V.F. Negrete. 1972. Doctor-patient communication. *Scientific American* 227: 66–74.

Kuczewski, M.G. 1996. Reconceiving the family: The process of consent in medical decision making. *Hastings Center Report* 26: 30–37.

Laforet, E.G. 1976. The fiction of informed consent. *Journal of the American Medical Association* 235 (15): 1579–85.

Lankton, J.W., B.M. Batchelder, and A.J. Ominsky. 1977. Emotional responses to detailed risk disclosure for anesthesia: A prospective, randomized study. *Anesthesiology* 46: 294–96.

Lavelle-Jones, C., D.J. Byrne, P. Rice, and A. Cushieri. 1993. Factors affecting quality of informed consent. *British Medical Journal* 306: 885–90.

Lazare, A., S. Eisenthal, and L. Wasserman. 1975. The customer approach to patienthood: Attending to patient requests in a walk-in clinic. *Archives of General Psychiatry* 32: 553–8.

Lee, P.P., J.C. Yang, and A.P. Schachat. 1993. Is informed consent needed for fluorescein angiography? *Archives of Ophthalmology* 111: 327–30.

Leeb, D., D.G. Bowers, and J.B. Lynch. 1976. Observations on the myth of informed consent. *Plastic Reconstructive Surgery* 58: 280–82.

Ley, P. 1983. Patients' understanding and recall in clinical communication failure. In *Doctor-patient communication*, edited by D. Pendleton and J. Hasler, 89–107. New York: Wiley and Sons.

Leydhecker, W., E. Gramer, and G.K. Krieglstein. 1980. Patient information before cataract surgery. *Ophthalmologica Base* 180: 241.

Lidz, C.W., A. Meisel, M. Osterweis, J.L. Holden, J.H. Marx, and M.R. Munetz. 1983. Barriers to informed consent. *Annals of Internal Medicine* 99: 539–43.

Lidz, C.W., A. Meisel, E. Zerubavel, M. Carter, R.M. Sestak, and L. Roth. 1984. *Informed consent: A study of decisionmaking in psychiatry.* New York: Guilford.

Lidz, C.W., P.S. Applebaum, and A. Meisel. 1988. Two models of implementing informed consent. *Archives of Internal Medicine* 148: 1385–89.

Lidz, C.W., and A. Meisel. 1982. Informed consent and the structure of medical care. In *Making health care decisions.* Vol. 2, 317–410. Washington, D.C.: U.S. President's Commission for the Study of Ethical Problems in Medicine and Biomedical and Behavioral Research.

Lidz, C.W., A. Meisel, and M. Munetz. 1985. Chronic disease: The sick role and informed consent. *Culture, Medicine and Psychiatry* 9: 241–55.

Lifton, R. J. 1986. *The nazi doctors.* New York: Basic Books.

Lippert, G.P., and D.E. Stewart. 1988. The psychiatrist's role in determining competency to consent in the general hospital. *Canadian Journal of Psychiatry* 33: 250–53.

Lo, B. 1990. Assessing decision-making capacity. *Law, Medicine and Health Care* 18: 192–201.

Lo, B., and G. McLeod. 1986. Patient attitudes to discussing life-sustaining treatment. *Archives of Internal Medicine* 146: 1613–15.

Loftus, E.F., and J.F. Fries. 1979. Informed consent may be hazardous to your health. *Science* 204: 11.

Lustig, A. 1996. Informed consent as a tool for medical management: A review by Stephen Wear. *Journal of Medicine and Philosophy* 21 (2): 101–9.

MacIntyre, A. 1981. *After virtue.* Notre Dame, Ind.: University of Notre Dame Press.

Maciunas, K.A., and A.H. Moss. 1992. Learning the patient's narrative to determine decision-making capacity: The role of ethics consultation. *Journal of Clinical Ethics* 3: 287–89.

Macklin, R. 1977. Consent, coercion, and conflicts of rights. *Perspectives in Biology and Medicine* 20: 360–71.

Mappes, T.A., and J.S. Zembaty. 1994. Patient choices, family interests, and physician obligations. *Kennedy Institute of Ethics Journal* 4: 27–46.

Mark, J.S., and H. Spiro. 1990. Informed consent for colonoscopy. *Archives of Internal Medicine* 150: 770–80.

Markham, B.B. 1975. The doctrine of informed consent—fact or fiction. *Forum* 10: 1073–79.

Marzuk, P.M. 1985. The right kind of paternalism. *New England Journal of Medicine* 313: 1474–76.

Mazur, D.J. 1986. What should patients be told prior to a medical procedure? Ethical and legal perspectives of medical informed consent. *American Journal of Medicine* 81 (6): 1051–54.

———. 1990. Judicial and legislative viewpoints on physician misestimation of patient dysutilities: A problem for decision analysts. *Medical Decision Making* 10: 172–80.

McCoid, A. 1957. A reappraisal of liability for unauthorized medical treatment. *Minnesota Law Review* 41: 381–434.

McCullough, L., and S. Wear. 1985. Respect for autonomy and medical paternalism reconsidered. *Theoretical Medicine* 6: 295–308.

McNeil, B.J. et al. 1982. On the elicitation of preferences for alternative therapies. *New England Journal of Medicine* 306: 1259.

Meichenbaum, D., and D. Turk. 1987. *Facilitating treatment adherence: A practitioner's guidebook.* New York: Plenum Press.

Meisel, A. 1979. The "exceptions" to the informed consent doctrine: Striking a balance between competing values in medical decisionmaking. *Wisconsin Law Review* 1979 (2): 413–88.

———. 1981. The "exceptions" to informed consent. *Connecticut Medicine* 45: 27–32.

———. 1988. A dignitary tort as a bridge between the idea of informed consent and the law of informed consent. *Law, Medicine and Health Care* 16 (3–4): 210–18.

Meisel, A., and L.H. Roth. 1981. What we do and do not know about informed consent. *Journal of the American Medical Association* 246: 2473–77.

———. 1983. Toward an informed discussion of informed consent: A review and critique of the empirical studies. *Arizona Law Review* 25: 265–346.

Merz, J.F., and B. Fischoff. 1990. Informed consent does not mean rational consent: Cognitive limitations on decision making. *Journal of Legal Medicine* 11 (3): 321–50.

Metro-Goldwyn-Mayer. 1981. *Whose life is it anyway?*

Miller, B.L. 1981. Autonomy and the refusal of lifesaving treatment. *Hastings Center Report* 11: 22–28.

Miller, R., and H.S. Willner. 1974. The two-part consent form: A suggestion for prompting free and informed consent. *New England Journal of Medicine* 290: 964–66.

Moreno, J.D. 1989. Treating the adolescent patient: An ethical analysis. *Journal of Adolescent Health Care* 10: 454–59.

———. 1994. Review of Stephen Wear's *Informed consent: Patient autonomy and physician beneficence in clinical medicine. Healthcare Ethics Committee Forum* 6 (5): 323–25.

Morgan, L.W., and I.R. Schwab. 1986. Informed consent for senile cataract extraction. *Archives of Ophthalmology* 104: 42–45.

Morreim, E.H. 1983. Three concepts of patient competence. *Theoretical Medicine* 4: 231–51.

———. 1986. Philosophy lessons from the clinical setting: Seven sayings that used to annoy me. *Theoretical Medicine* 7: 47–63.

———. 1991. Competence: At the intersection of law, medicine and philosophy. In *Competency: A study of informal competency determinations in primary care,* edited by M.A. Gardell and E. Shelp, 93–125. Dordrecht, Netherlands: Kluwer Academic Publishers.

———. 1995. *Balancing act: The new medical ethics of medicine's new economics.* Washington, D.C.: Georgetown University Press.

Morrow, G.R. 1980. How readable are subject consent forms? *Journal of the American Medical Association* 244: 56–58.

Morrow, G., R. Gootnick, and A. Schmale. 1978. A simple technique for increasing cancer patients' knowledge of informed consent to treatment. *Cancer* 42: 793–99.

Murphy, D.J., D. Burrows, S. Santilli et al. 1994. The influence of the probability of survival on patients' preferences regarding cardiopulmonary resuscitation. *New England Journal of Medicine* 330 (8): 545–49.

Murphy, J. 1974. Incompetence and paternalism. *Archiv für Rechts-und-Sozialphilosophie* 50: 465–86.

———. 1979. Therapy and the problem of autonomous consent. *International Journal of Law and Psychiatry* 2: 415–30.

Murray, C. 1984. *Losing ground*. New York: Basic Books.

Nathanson, V. 1996. Review of Stephen Wear's *Informed consent: Patient autonomy and physician beneficence in clinical medicine. International Digest of Health Legislation* 47 (2): 273–75.

Novack, P. et al. 1979. Physicians' attitudes toward telling the cancer patient. *Journal of the American Medical Association* 241: 897.

Nuland, S.B. 1994. *How we die: Reflections on life's final chapter*. New York: Knopf.

Oberst, M. 1984. Patients' perceptions of care: Measurement of quality and satisfaction. *Cancer* 53: 2366–73.

Office of Technology Assessment. 1987. *Life-sustaining technologies and the elderly*. Washington, D.C.: Congress of the United States.

O'Hair, D. 1986. Patient preferences for physician persuasion strategies. *Theoretical Medicine* 7: 147–64.

Oken, D. 1961. What to tell cancer patients: A study of medical attitudes. *Journal of the American Medical Association* 175: 1120.

O'Neill, O. 1984. Paternalism and partial autonomy. *Journal of Medical Ethics* 10: 173–78.

Ozar, D. 1984. "Patients" autonomy: Three models of the professional-lay relationship in medicine. *Theoretical Medicine* 5: 61–68.

Parsons, T. 1975. The sick role and the role of the physician considered. *Milbank Memorial Fund Quarterly* 53: 257–77.

Pasek, J. 1995. Review of Stephen Wear's *Informed consent: Patient autonomy and physician beneficence in clinical medicine. Journal of Medical Ethics* 21 (2): 119–20.

Peabody, F.W. 1927. The care of the patient. *Journal of the American Medical Association* 88: 877–82.

Pellegrino, E.D. 1979. Toward a reconstruction of medical morality: The primacy of the act of profession and the fact of illness. *Journal of Medicine and Philosophy* 4: 35–46.

Pellegrino, E.D., and D.C. Thomasma. 1981. *A philosophical basis of medical practice*. Oxford, New York: Oxford University Press.

———. 1988. *For the patient's good: The restoration of beneficence in health care*. New York: Oxford University Press.

Pendleton, D.A., and S. Bochner. 1980. The communication of medical information in general practice consultations as a function of patient's social class. *Social Science in Medicine* 14: 669–73.

Perl, M., and E.E. Shelp. 1982. Psychiatric consultation masking moral dilemmas in medicine. *New England Journal of Medicine* 307: 618–21.

Pernick, M. 1982. The patient's role in medical decision-making: A social history of informed consent in medical therapy. In *Making health care decisions. The ethical and legal implications of informed consent in the patient-practitioner relationship*, compiled by the President's Commission for the Study of Ethical Problems in Medicine and Biomedical and Behavioral Research. Vol. 2, of informed consent, 1–35. Washington, D.C.: U.S. Government Printing Office.

Perry, C.B., and W.B. Applegate. 1985. Medical paternalism and patient self-determination. *Journal of the American Geriatric Society* 33: 353–59.

President's Commission for the Study of Ethical Problems in Medicine and Biomedical and Behavioral Research, comp. 1982. *Making health care decisions: The ethical and legal implications of informed consent in the patient-practitioner relationship*. Washington, D.C.: U.S. Government Printing Office.

———. 1983. *Deciding to forego life sustaining treatment: Ethical, medical and legal issues in treatment decisions*. Washington, D.C.: U.S. Government Printing Office.

Priluck, I.A., D.M. Robertson, and H. Buettner. 1979. What patients recall of the preoperative discussion after retinal detachment surgery. *American Journal of Ophthalmology* 87: 620–63.

Quill, T.E. 1983. Partnerships in patient care: A contractual approach. *Annals of Internal Medicine* 98: 228–34.

Quill, T.E., and H. Brody. 1996. Physician recommendations and patient autonomy: Finding a balance between physician power and patient choice. *Annals of Internal Medicine* 125: 763–69.

Quill, T.E., and P. Townsend. 1991. Bad news: Delivery, dialogue, and dilemmas. *Archives of Internal Medicine* 151: 463–68.

Ramsey, P. 1970. *The patient as person*. New Haven, Conn.: Yale University Press.

Rasinski, Dorothy C. 1993. Cross-cultural concerns and communication in health care. In *Perspectives on Health Communication*, edited by B.C. Thornton and G.L. Kreps, 165–77, New York: Waveland Press.

Ravitch, M. 1978. The myth of informed consent. *Surgical Rounds* 1: 7–8.

Reiser, S.J. 1980. Words as scalpels: Transmitting evidence in the clinical dialogue. *Annals of Internal Medicine* 92: 837–42.

Rennie, D. 1980. Informed consent by well-nigh abject adults. *New England Journal of Medicine* 302: 917–18.

Robinson, G., and A. Merav. 1976. Informed consent: Recall by patients tested postoperatively. *Annals of Thoracic Surgery* 22: 209–12.

Rosenberg, H. 1973. Informed consent: A reappraisal of patients' reactions. *California Medicine* 119: 64–68.

Roth, L.H. et al. 1977. Tests of competency to consent to treatment. *American Journal of Psychiatry* 134: 279–84.

Roth, L., and A. Meisel. 1981. What we do and do not know about informed consent. *Journal of the American Medical Association* 246: 2473–77.

Roth, L., A. Meisel, and C.W. Lidz. 1982. The dilemma of denial in the assessment of competency to refuse treatment. *American Journal of Psychiatry* 139: 910–13.

Rothman, D.J. 1991. *Strangers at the bedside*. New York: Basic Books.

Rozovsky, F.A. 1984. *Consent to treatment: A practical guide*. Boston: Little, Brown.

Ryan, R.M. 1993. Agency and organization: Intrinsic motivation, autonomy and the self in pyschological development. Nebraska Symposium on Motivation Current Theory and Research. In *Motivation*, 1–56. Lincoln: University of Nebraska Press.

Ryan, R.M., E.L. Deci, and W.S. Grolnick. 1995. Autonomy, relatedness and the self: Their relation to development and pyschopathology. In *Developmental psychopathology*, edited by D. Cicchetti and D.J. Cohen, 618–55. New York: Wiley.

Sbarbaro, J.A. 1990. The patient-physician relationship: Compliance revisited. *Annals of Allergy* 64: 325–31.

Schneiderman, L.J., and J.D. Arras. 1985. Counseling patients to counsel physicians on future care in the event of patient incompetence. *Annals of Internal Medicine* 102: 693–98.

Schneiderman, L.J., R.M. Kaplan, R.A. Pearlman, and H. Teezel. 1993. Do physicians' own preferences for life-sustaining treatment influence their perceptions of patients' preferences? *Journal of Clinical Ethics* 4: 28–33.

Schoene-Seifert, B., and J.F. Childress. 1986. How much should the cancer patient know and decide? *CA-A Cancer Journal for Clinicians* 36 (2): 85–94.

Schwartz, R., and A. Grubb. 1985. Why Britain can't afford informed consent. *Hastings Center Report* 15: 20.

Sharp, M.C., R.P. Strauss, and S.C. Lorch. 1992. Communicating medical bad news. Parents' experiences and preferences. *Journal of Pediatrics* 121: 539–46.

Shelp, E.E. 1985. *Virtue and medicine*. Boston: Reidel.

———. 1986. *Born to die?: Deciding the fate of critically ill newborns*. New York: Free Press.

Shelp, E.E., and M. Perl. 1985. Denial in clinical medicine. *Archives of Internal Medicine* 145: 697–99.

Sherlock, R. 1983. Consent, competency and ECT: Some critical suggestions. *Journal of Medical Ethics* 9: 141–43.

———. 1984. Competency to consent to medical care: Toward a general view. *General Hospital Psychiatry* 6: 71–76.

Shertzer, M. 1986. *The elements of grammar*. New York: Collier Books/Macmillan.

Shimm, D.S., and Roy G. Spece, Jr. 1991. Conflict of interest and informed consent in industry-sponsored clinical trials. *Journal of Legal Medicine* 12: 477–513.

Siegler, M. 1977. Critical illness: The limits of autonomy. *Hastings Center Report* 7: 12–15.

————. 1982. Decision making strategy for clinical-ethical problems in medicine. *Archives of Internal Medicine* 142: 2179.

————. 1993. Falling off the pedestal: What is happening to the traditional doctor-patient relationship? *Mayo Clinic Proceedings* 68: 461–67.

Simnoff, L.A., and J.H. Fetting. 1991. Factors affecting treatment decisions for a life threatening illness: The case of medical treatment of breast cancer. *Social Science and Medicine* 32 (7): 813–18.

Sprung, C.L., and B.J. Winnick. 1989. Informed consent theory and practice. *CriticalCare Medicine* 17: 1346–54.

Smith, D.H. 1992. Stories, values, and patient care decision making. In *The ethical nexus: Value, communication and organizational decision*, edited by C. Conrad, 8–23. Norwood, N.J.: Ablex.

Smith, D.H., and L. Newton. 1984. Physician and patient: Respect for mutuality. *Theoretical Medicine* 5: 43–60.

Smith, D.H., and R.B. Hope. 1991. The patient's story: Integrating the patient and physician-centered approaches to interviewing. *Annals of Internal Medicine* 115: 470–77.

Squier, R.W. 1990. A model of empathic understanding and adherence to treatment regimens in practitioner-patient relationships. *Social Science and Medicine* 30: 325–39.

Stagno, S.J., M.L. Smith, and S.J. Hassenbusch. 1994. Reconsidering "psychosurgery": Issues of informed consent and physician responsibility. *Journal of Clinical Ethics* 5 (3): 217–23.

Stanley, B., J. Guido, M. Stanley, D. Shortell. 1984. The elderly patient and informed consent: Empirical findings. *Journal of the American Medical Association* 252 (10): 1302–6.

Starr, P. 1982. *The social transformation of American medicine*. New York: Basic Books.

Strong, C. 1993. Patients should not always come first in treatment decisions. *Journal of Clinical Ethics* 4: 63–75.

Strub, R.L., and F.W. Black. 1977. *The mental status examination in neurology*. Philadelphia: F. A. Davis.

Strull, W.M. et al. 1985. Do patients want to participate in medical decision making? *Journal of the American Medical Association* 252: 2990–94.

Szasz, T.S., and M. Hollender. 1956. The basic models of the doctor-patient relationship. *Archives of Internal Medicine* 97: 585–92.

Szasz, T.S. 1961. *The myth of mental illness*. New York: Hoeber-Harper.

Szczygiel, A. 1994. Beyond informed consent. *Ohio Northern University Law Review* 21: 171–262.

Tait, K., and G. Winslow. 1977. Beyond consent: The ethics of decision-making in emergency medicine. *Western Journal of Medicine* 126: 158.

Tancredi, L. 1982. Competency for informed consent. *International Journal of Law and Psychiatry* 5: 51–63.

Taub, S. 1982. Cancer and the law of informed consent. *Law, Medicine and Health Care* 10: 61.

Thomasma, D.C. 1983a. Beyond medical paternalism and patient autonomy. *Annals of Internal Medicine* 98: 243–48.

———. 1983b. Limitations of the autonomy model for the doctor-patient relationship. *Pharos* 46: 2–5.

———. 1994. Models for the doctor-patient relationship and the ethics committees, II. *Cambridge Quarterly of Healthcare Ethics* 3: 10–26.

Treffert, D. 1974. Dying with your rights on. *Prism* 2: 49–52.

Uhlmann, R.F., R.A. Pearlman, and K.C. Cain. 1988. Physicians' and spouses' predictions of elderly patients' resuscitation preferences. *Journal of Gerontology* 43: 115–21.

Veatch, R.M. 1972. Medical ethics: Professional or universal? *Harvard Theological Review* 65: 531–59.

———. 1974. Models for ethical medicine in a revolutionary age. *Hastings Center Report* 2: 5–7.

———. 1981. *A theory of medical ethics*. New York Basic Books.

———. 1991. *The patient-physician relationship: The patient as partner*. Bloomington: Indiana University Press.

Videotape "Please Let Me Die" in the Library of Psychiatric Disorders series. 1974. Department of Psychiatry, University of Texas Medical Branch at Galveston.

Wagner, A. 1985. Cardiopulmonary resuscitation in the aged: A prospective study. *New England Journal of Medicine* 310: 1129–30.

Waitzkin, H. 1984. Doctor-patient communication: Clinical implications of social scientific research. *Journal of the American Medical Association* 252 (17): 2441–46.

Waitzkin, H., and J. Stoeckle. 1976. Information control and the micro-politics of health care: Summary of an ongoing research project. *Social Science and Medicine* 10: 263–76.

Wallace, L.M. 1986. Informed consent to elective surgery: The therapeutic value. *Social Science and Medicine* 22: 29–33.

Wanzer, S., D.D. Federman, S.J. Adelstein, C.K. Cassel, E.H. Cassem, R.E. Crawford, E.W. Hook, B. Lo, C.G. Moertel, P. Safar, A. Stone, and J.V. Eys. 1984. The physician's responsibility toward hopelessly ill patients. *New England Journal of Medicine* 310: 955–59.

Wanzer, S., D.D. Federman, S.J. Adelstein, C.K. Cassel, E.H. Cassem, R.E. Crawford, E.W. Hook, B. Lo, C.G. Moertel, P. Safar, A. Stone, and J.V. Eys. 1989. The physician's responsibility toward hopelessly ill patients: A second look. *New England Journal of Medicine* 320: 844–49.

Wear, S. 1979. The diminished moral status of the mentally ill. In *Mental illness: Law and public policy*, edited by B. Brody et al., 221–30. Dordrecht, Netherlands: Reidel.

———. 1980. Mental illness and moral status. *Journal of Medicine and Philosophy* 5: 292–312.

———. 1983. Patient autonomy, paternalism, and the conscientious physician. *Theoretical Medicine* 4: 253–74.

———. 1987. Review of Richard Zaner's *Ethics and the clinical encounter*. *American Philosophical Association Newsletter on Philosophy and Medicine* 88: 40–42.

————. 1989. Anticipatory ethical decision-making: The role of the primary physician. *HMO Practice* 3: 41–46.

————. 1991. Patient freedom and competence in health care. In *Competency: A study of informal competency determinations in primary care*, edited by M.A.G. Cutter and E.E. Shelp, 227–36. Dordrecht, Netherlands: Kluwer Academic Publishers.

Wear, S., P. Katz, B. Andrezjewski, and T. Haryadi. 1990. The development of an ethics consultation service. *Hospital Ethics Committee Forum* 2: 75–87.

Weinstein, M.C. et al. 1980: *Clinical decision analysis*. Philadelphia: Saunders.

Weiss, G.B. 1985. Paternalism modernized. *Journal of Medical Ethics* 11: 184–87.

Weithorn, L.A., and S.B. Campbell. 1982. The competency of children and adolescents to make informed treatment decisions. *Child Development* 53: 1589.

Wikler, D. 1979. Paternalism and the mildly retarded. *Philosophy and Public Affairs* 8: 377–421.

Wolf, A., J.F. Nasser, A.M. Wolf, and J.B. Schorling. 1996. The impact of informed consent on patient interest in prostrate-specific antigen screening. *Archives of Internal Medicine* 156: 1333–36.

Wolf, S.M. 1994. Health care reform and the future of the physician ethics. *Hastings Center Report* 24: 28–41.

Zaner, R. 1988. *Ethics and the clinical encounter*. Englewood Cliffs, N.J.: Prentice Hall.

Index